Scope® Monograph on

PATHOPARASITOLOGY

A color atlas of parasites in tissue sections

MICHAEL KENNEY M.D., D.T.M., F.C.A.P.

Professor of Pathology, State University of New York, Downstate Medical Center
Chief, Tropical Disease and Parasitology Service,
Kings County Hospital, Institute of Pathology, Brooklyn, N.Y.

PUBLISHED BY THE UPJOHN COMPANY, KALAMAZOO, MICHIGAN

Editor/ Baird A. Thomas

Library of Congress Card Number 72-79694

Reprinted 1974
⋹ S-2835R

Contents

Preface

This monograph of Pathoparasitology, a color atlas of parasites in tissue sections, is primarily intended as a guide for medical students interested in pathology and parasitology. Its purpose is to assist beginners, already engaged in diagnostic pathology, who are finding parasites with increasing frequency in both surgical and autopsy material. Constantly growing world travel to endemic areas, increasing pollution of the environment, overpopulation leading to poorer personal hygiene, are just a few examples of the multiple causes contributing to the spread of parasitic infections, which already are major medical and public health problems.

This monograph is not intended for the review of either basic pathology or parasitology. Therefore, detailed description of tissues and their reactions to parasitic invasion, and the detailed morphological study of parasites with their life cycles, were not included. However, the important criteria for recognition of parasites and for their differential diagnosis in tissue sections are stressed.

In order to make the monograph practical, the material has been oriented by *body systems* and not by the classification of parasites. To assist those who might refer to a particular organ, some duplication of parasites could not be avoided. However, different aspects of sectioned parasites are presented in such cases. For the same purpose, no attempt was made to include spectacular illustrations but rather those aspects of parasites which are usually observed in routine tissue sections.

Almost all of the tissue sections from which the illustrations were made were stained with hematoxylin-eosin. This method has been selected because it is the usual technique used in every histopathology laboratory, thus familiarizing a student of pathology with the picture of parasites encountered in routine material. However, occasionally sections stained by special staining methods are presented to stress the advantage of such methods in certain cases. All illustrations can be considered to be hematoxylin-eosin stained sections except those otherwise labeled. The variation in color of illustrations representing tissue sections stained with hematoxylin-eosin are due to many factors, such as technical differences in various histopathology laboratories in which the sections had been processed and the variation in original Kodachrome prints made from transparencies.

All magnifications listed are those used in taking the photomicrographs. However, for uniformity, all illustrations have been made the same size.

Because of limited space and number of color illustrations of this monograph, it did not seem indicated to include extremely rare, accidentally-human parasites, which a physician would probably never encounter during his whole career. On the other hand, some of the more common parasites have been presented in greater detail. In fact, the two-dimentional tissue section may pass through any part of the parasite and sectioning at various angles gives multiple aspects of the same parasite. Furthermore, old infections, followed by degeneration and calcification of the parasite and the tissue of the host, add more difficulties to the diagnostic problems inherent in the nature of tissue sections.

All illustrations in this monograph were produced from Kodachrome slides I have made personally. With rare exceptions the transparencies had been made from tissue section slides in my teaching collection. The original material, an accumulation of many decades, came from various sources, and, in most cases, it was not possible to trace its origin for proper credit. However, I wish to acknowledge all possible sources of this material.

My deep gratitude is due to:

Harold W. Brown, M.D., Professor Emeritus of Parasitology and Dr. Kathleen L. Hussey, Professor of Parasitology, Columbia University, School of Public Health and Administrative Medicine, New York, who for many years had generously shared with me the material from their personal collections, their knowledge and experience.

Stanley M. Aronson, M.D., Professor and Chairman, Department of Pathology, Brown University, Providence, Rhode Island, for tissue sections given me from both the services he now directs and while he was Professor of Pathology, State University of New York, Downstate Medical Center, and Director, Kings County Hospital, Institute of Pathology, Brooklyn, N.Y.

Valentin Yermakov, M.D., Assoc. Professor of Pathology, State University of New York, Downstate Medical Center, and Director, Kings County Hospital, Institute of Pathology, Brooklyn, N.Y., and his staff, for making available to me all autopsy and surgical pathology material containing parasites.

Cassius Plair, M.D., Chief, Anatomical Pathology Section, Laboratory Service, Veterans Administration Hospital, New York who during many years of our association had never failed to bring to my atttention tissue sections with parasites.

Dr. G. B. Solomon, Assistant Professor, University of Pennsylvania, The School of Veterinary Medicine, for providing me with tissue sections with *Capillaria hepatica.*

Lorenz E. Zimmerman, M.D., Chief Ophthalmic Pathology Branch, Armed Forces Institute of Pathology, Washington, D.C., for making available to me sections of visceral larva migrans in the retina.

Sidney C. Kress, Major, USAF, MC, Malcolm USAF Medical Center, Andrews AFB., Washington, D.C., for the lung tissue section with the larval form of *Linguatula serrata.*

Parasitology Section, National Communicable Disease Center, Atlanta, Georgia for the lung tissue sections with *Pneumocystis carinii.*

Students and residents participating in my teaching seminars, who, busy with their new assignments elsewhere, remembered and found time to bring me material they knew I would want to add to my collection.

My colleagues in the then Belgian Congo and British Guiana, whose names I now cannot remember, but whose generosity many decades ago allowed me to start my teaching collection.

Other tissue sections which might have been used in making the Kodachromes could have originated from The Armed Forces Institute of Pathology, Washington, D.C., Carolina Biological Supply Company, Burlington, North Carolina, and Ward's Natural Science Extablishment, Inc., Rochester, New York.

I wish to express my warm gratitude to my wife, Lona B. Kenney, author in her own right, whose help and encouragement enabled me to complete this monograph.

And last, but not least, I am very glad to have the opportunity to thank the publishers and Mr. B. A. Thomas, the editor. Through the medium of this monograph they have allowed me to enter once more the vast auditorium of the world and face new young students and residents wanting to learn what I have to offer them.

Intestine

The intestinal tract is the site of numerous parasites belonging to both groups, the protozoa, i.e., unicellular organisms detectable only with the help of a microscope, and metazoa, the multicellular organisms. The latter include such large parasites as the tapeworm, which sometimes measure over ten meters in length. However, only a few of the intestinal parasites actually penetrate, or are attached to, the mucosal lining of the intestinal wall, and can be found in tissue sections.

Occasionally, some parasites, both pathogenic and nonpathogenic, which normally live in the lumen of the intestinal tract, are sectioned together with the tissue thus establishing the diagnosis of an often unsuspected parasitic infection. This is even more frequent in sections of the appendix which, because of its natural configuration, acts as a trap for the parasites. The histopathologic sections of the appendix often keep their contents, while the contents of the small and large intestines are often lost during the process of fixation, sectioning and staining. When a parasite, its egg, or cyst are found in the appendix, it frequently comes from the large intestine where the parasite lives, e.g., *Trichuris trichiura* (whipworm), or *Enterobius vermicularis* (pinworm, seatworm). Rarely is it a parasite which because of its erratic nature may wander out of the small intestine and get trapped in the appendix, e.g., *Ascaris lumbricoides* (roundworm). Sometimes a parasite which may invade the mucosa is observed in the lumen of the appendix before it has had a chance to establish itself in the tissue. In addition to the parasites in the intestinal tract, others may invade the mesentery, e.g., the schistosomes and the hydatid cyst of *Echinococcus granulosus.*

Entamoeba histolytica

The diagnosis of amebiasis due to *E. histolytica* may appear easier in tissue sections than in stool examinations. Among the five species of human amebae found in the large intestine *(Entamoeba histolytica, Entamoeba coli, Iodamoeba butschlii, Endolimax nana,* and *Dientamoeba fragilis),* only *E. histolytica* is believed to be able to penetrate and destroy the intestinal mucosa and submucosa. Although recent investigations point to the possibility that pathogenic strains of soil-water amebae causing meningoencephalitis in man may invade other tissues, for all practical purposes, the only differential diagnosis between an ameba found in the tissue of the large intestine is between *E. histolytica* and a large macrophage. The latter can be ruled out by the presence of its comparatively large nucleus which appears in a section as a dark, irregular mass, unlike the nucleus of *E. histolytica.* In some instances, there may be no visible nucleus in *E. histolytica,* which seldom occurs in a sectioned macrophage.

The lesions produced by *E. histolytica* are frequently found in the cecum, ascending colon and sigmoidorectal region. However, the primary site may also be found in other areas including the terminal portion of the ileum and the appendix. The lesions may progress from early, round or oval, minute ulcerations affecting the mucosal lining to deep, necrotic destruction of the intestinal wall.

The diagnostic features of *E. histolytica* are its characteristic nucleus with its minute, delicate central karyosome, and a very uniformly stained ring of peripheral chromatin of even thickness. However, this pathognomonic picture, which is easily detectable in stained smears, is often absent in tissue sections. In fact, the nucleus of an ameba is relatively small and the tissue sections are thin enough to bypass it most of the time. A secondary diagnostic feature of *E. histolytica,* the presence of erythrocytes in the cytoplasm of the large pathogenic strain, may not be observed after the amebae have invaded the tissue. On the contrary, another diagnostic feature never observed in the smears but always found in the tissue sections is histolysis of the invaded tissue, i.e., a clear zone around the ameba. Although the consensus is that *E. histolytica* may be found in tissues only in its trophozoite stage, there is evidence that under certain conditions it may form cysts within the invaded tissue. Such cystic forms may have one to four nuclei and also contain cigar-shaped chromatoidal bodies.

Balantidium coli

B. coli, the only pathogenic ciliate of man, is the natural parasite of the pig. However, incidental human infections with this large protozoon, measuring up to 150 microns by 120 microns (average 60/45 microns), may be quite severe. Pathologic changes may range from simple catharal hyperemia of the mucosa to marked ulcerations produced by both active penetration and cytolytic ferments secreted by the parasite. Although the predilection of *B. coli* is the cecum, where the infection often results in abscess formation, balantidiasis has also been found in other portions of the large bowel, including the appendix.

Enterobius vermicularis (pinworm, seatworm)

This small nematode, measuring 2-13mm. in length, is a cosmopolitan parasite with a world-wide distribution. Man is its only known host. The usual

Fig. 1. Amebiasis of the colon.
A section of the colon demonstrates part of a typical flask-shaped amebic ulcer. The mucosa is destroyed only on the right side but the lesion extends laterally and in depth under the undermined mucosa. Even at low magnification one can see pinpoint amebae (A) in the deep layers of yet unsloughed, but already affected, mucosa in the center of the illustration. (x35)

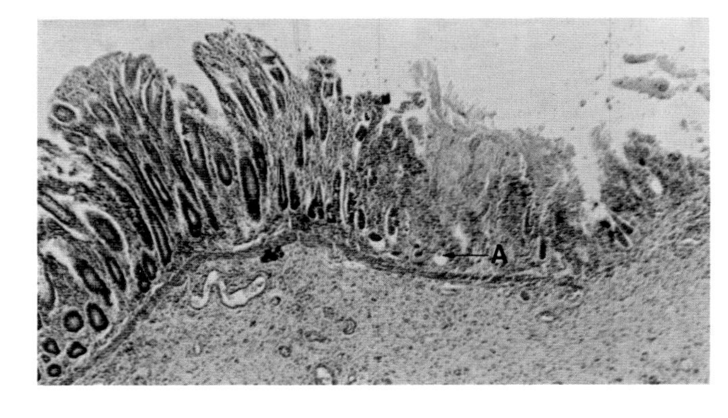

Fig. 2. Entamoeba histolytica in the large intestine.
The examination of the mucosa of the large intestine reveals the presence of *E. histolytica (E.h.).* The irregular mottled ameba in the center of the illustration demonstrates a nucleus (N) with its central karyosome (K) and peripheral ring of chromatin (C). There is a clear space around the ameba, the result of histolysis of the tissue, characteristic of *E. histolytical* infection. (x400)

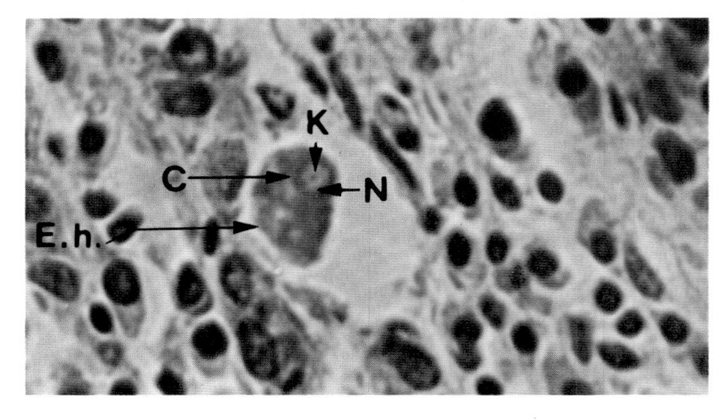

Fig. 3. *Balantidium coli* in the large intestine.
Even at low magnification, numerous *B. coli* (B.c.) can be recognized in the deep portion of the submucosa of the large intestine. The protozoa are much larger than the pinpoint cells of inflammatory origin near the mucosa. (x35)

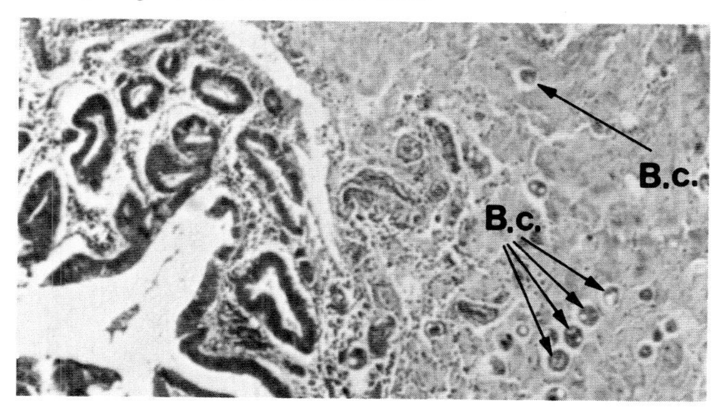

Fig. 4. *Balantidium coli* in the appendix.
Section of the appendix demonstrates numerous *B. coli* (B.c.) invading the mucosa. Some of the protozoa show the typical kidney-shaped nucleus (N), large contractile vacuoles (V) left, and peripheral cilia (C). There are hemorrhagic areas and irregular oval ulcers with communicating sinuses which replace the normal architecture of the mucosa in an advanced case of balantidiasis. Cellular reaction at this stage is minimal. (x400)

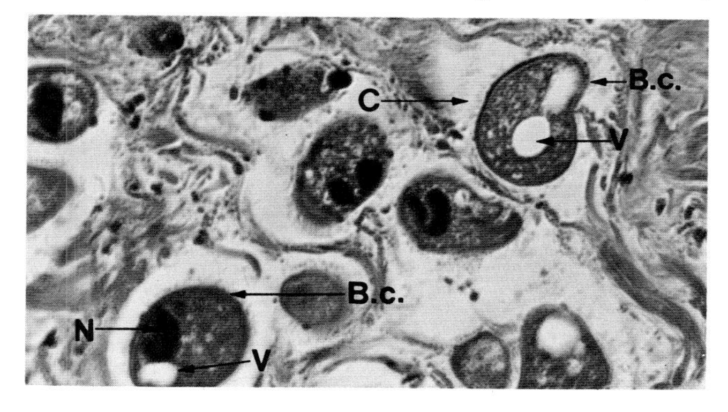

Fig. 5. *Enterobius vermicularis* in the appendix.
A cross-section of *E. vermicularis* (E.v.) in the lumen of the appendix. Note two minute triangular alae (A), diagnotic for this species, situated externally on opposite sides of the parasite. Beneath the cuticle (C) of the nematode, the wall formed by the muscle fibers (MF) is of meromyerial type, i.e., containing relatively few muscle fibers of varying size. (x100)

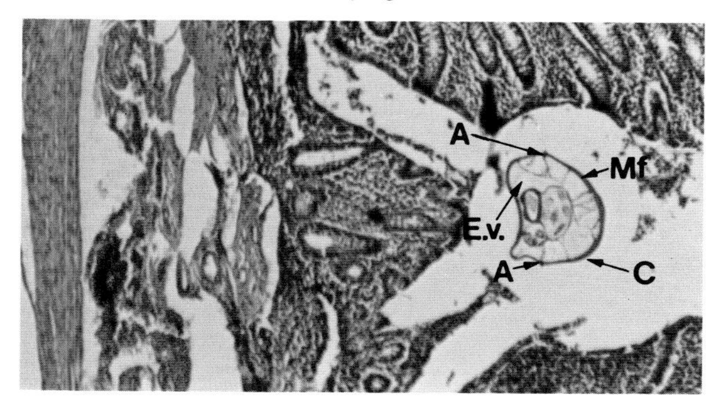

habitat of *E. vermicularis* is the cecum and frequently the appendix. However, immature males and females may be found in the lower part of the ileum, rectum and occasionally up in the stomach. The gravid female has its nocturnal migration to the perianal regions for oviposition. The diagnosis of *E. vermicularis* in tissue sections is faciliated by the presence of cuticular wing-like expansions, which are more prominent at the anterior end of the parasite, but continue bilaterally all the way to the posterior extremity. These alae appear on all cross-sections of the pinworm as minute triangles situated externally on two opposite sides of the worm. *E. vermicularis* does not attach to the intestinal mucosa and lesions are unusual in tissue sections. However, wandering females have been reported accidentally migrating into the urethra, the urinary bladder, vagina, fallopian tubes and into the peritoneal cavity. Autoinfection in enterobiasis is common as the eggs become infectious shortly after being laid around the anus, producing an irritation and inducing scratching.

Ascaris lumbricoides (roundworm)

This large nematode, measuring 10-35cm., is a cosmopolitan parasite, prominent in the tropics. Like many other human parasites, its frequency of infection is related to overcrowding and poor sanitary conditions. *A. lumbricoides* usually lives in the small intestine but because of its erratic nature it often migrates far from its natural habitat. This migration is often due to unrelated fever or to drugs taken by the host which irritate but do not have a lethal effect on the worm. Complications that may arise from such wanderings range in severity from simple regurgitation and vomiting of the worm, to more severe invasion of the bile ducts, the liver, and even the abdominal cavity by active perforation of the intestinal wall which may result in fatal peritonitis. Obstruction of the appendix is perhaps one of the most frequent complications in severe infection. Because of its large size and tapering ends it is the anterior part of the *Ascaris* which is most often found in an obstructed appendix although occasionally ova of an *Ascaris* are found in a tissue section of the appendix. These eggs may be either fertile or infertile. An infertile *Ascaris* egg is readily recognized by its mammillated covering which is flatter than that on fertilized eggs, its relatively narrow form but larger size (88-94/39-44 microns) as compared to the size of fertilized eggs (45-70/35-50 microns). An infertile egg does not necessarily suggest the absence of male worms in the intestine but rather a smaller number of parasites. A single female has a daily output of about 200,000 eggs and

Fig. 6. Ascaris lumbricoides in the appendix.

The anterior end of *A. lumbriocoides* (A.l.) in cross section fills the lumen of the appendix. At this level the tissue section shows only the central flattened digestive tract (DT) of the parasite and the peripheral muscular wall under the external cuticle. The muscle fibers (MF) are of polymyerial type, i.e., irregular, very long, and penetrate deeply into the body cavity of the parasite. These muscle fibers are considerably longer than the thickness of the external cuticle (C). (x12)

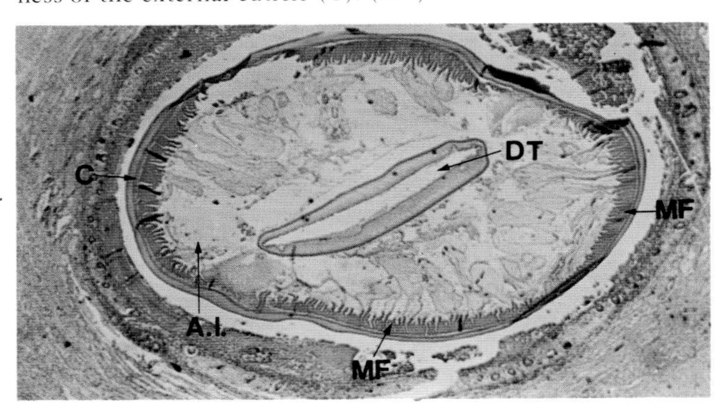

Fig. 7. Ascaris lumbriocoides in the appendix.

Part of *A. lumbricoides* in a cross-section of the appendix, under higher magnification. Under the external smooth cuticle (C) is the wall formed by very long but uneven muscle fibers (MF) of polymyerial type which extends deep into the body cavity of the roundworm. Left of the parasite is hemorrhagic inflammatory exudate (IE). (x400)

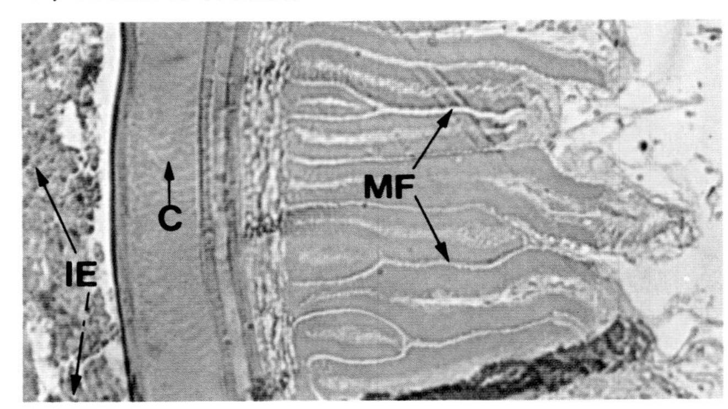

Fig. 8. Trichuris trichiura in the appendix.

A characteristic picture of *T. trichiura* in a cross-section of the appendix. The thick body (B) and above and slightly to the right, the thin "whip" (W) portion of the parasite can be seen. DT is the digestive tract. (x40)

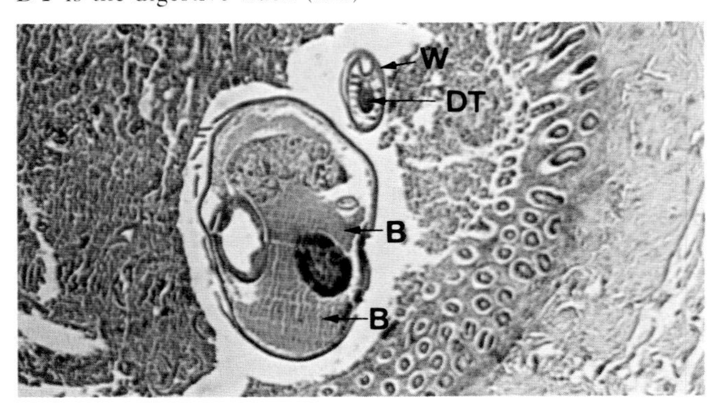

Fig. 9. Trichuris trichiura in the appendix.

The cross-section of *T. trichiura* (T.t.) demonstrates, under high magnification, the smooth outside cuticle (C) and the evenly low, tightly packed, relatively short muscle fibers (MF) of holomyerial type. Appendix (Ap) tissue is seen above the parasite. (x400)

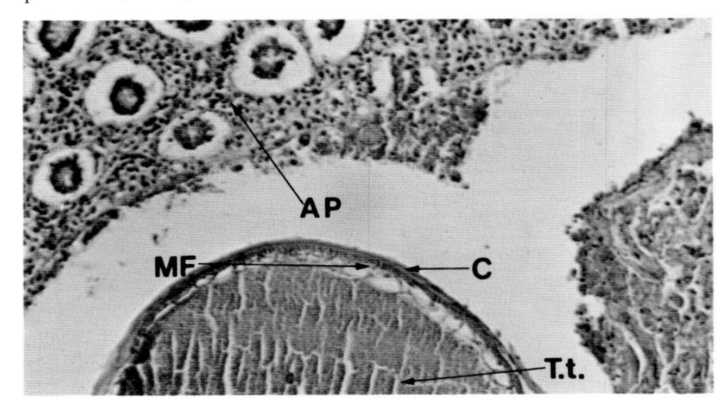

repeated copulation with a male is necessary to fertilize them all. *Ascaris* because of its complex life cycle may also be found in tissue sections in its larval stage.

In sections, *Ascaris* can be recognized by its large size and its characteristic muscular wall of polymyerial type, i.e., formed by very long, irregular muscle fibers.

Trichuris trichiura (whipworm)

This nematode is a natural parasite of the large intestine of man. It has a peculiar morphology which facilitates its recognition in tissue sections. Less than half of its total length of 30-50mm. consists of a thick posterior body and the rest by an attenuated, whip-like anterior portion. Because the long worm is often folded on itself, more so in the narrow lumen of the appendix, most sections reveal both the robust body and the slender anterior end. The muscular wall under the cuticle of *Trichuris* is of holomyerial type characterized by evenly low, tightly packed, relatively short muscle fibers. The recognition of this type of musculature is important for diagnosis when the body section of the parasite is not accompanied by a section of the "whip," the thin anterior portion.

In slight infections no inflammatory reaction is usually incited. In heavy infections, however, hemorrhages, subacute inflammatory changes, and evidence of secondary bacterial contamination may be found at the site of penetration by the "whips," occasionally resulting in peritonitis.

The female of *T. trichiura* deposits from 3,000 to 10,000 eggs daily. Since the worm has a predilection for the cecum, it is not infrequent to find whipworm eggs in sections of the appendix, thus establishing the diagnosis of active trichuriasis. Such a diagnosis is easy when the eggs are sectioned longitudinally. They are usually golden-brown, 50-54 microns in length, and have a characteristic lemon-shaped form with two plug-like polar structures. The diagnosis of an occasional cross-sectioned egg of *T. trichiura* in the appendix is more difficult. The brown color of the egg and its diameter of 23 microns are often used as diagnostic criteria in such cases. However, recent studies show that the size and color of *Trichuris* eggs can vary readily, especially in debilitated children.

Intestinal myiasis

The possibility of a true intestinal myiasis, i.e., the development of maggots of flies in the intestinal mucosa of man, has been discussed for decades. Intestinal myiasis does exist in animals, e.g., *Gasterophilus*, a parasite of the alimentary canal of horses

Fig. 10. Trichuris trichiura in the appendix.
The cross-section of the anterior "whip" (W) portion of *T. trichiura* demonstrates its characteristic smooth outside cuticle (C), the even, tightly packed muscular wall of holomyerial type, and the central esophagus (E). (x20)

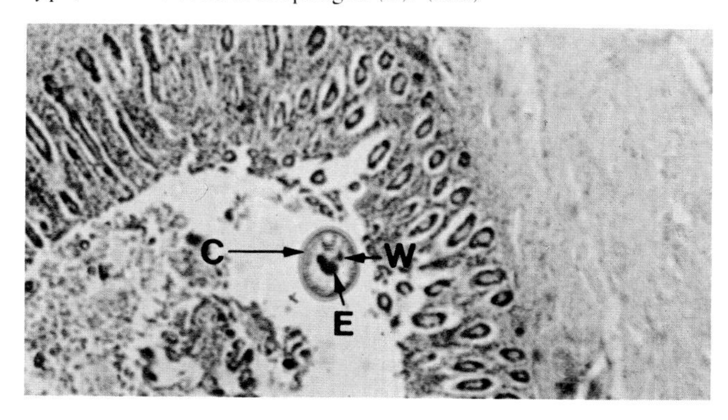

Fig. 11. Ova of *Trichuris trichiura* in the appendix.
There are numerous eggs (E) of *T. trichiura* in this section. Some of the eggs are sectioned longitudinally and demonstrate their characteristic lemon-shaped form and the plug-like polar structures (P). Occasional eggs contain elongated developing larvae (L), top right. Eggs of this species are usually found in unsegmented stage, the presence of eggs with embryonic development in the appendix indicates prolonged stagnation of fecal contents. (x100)

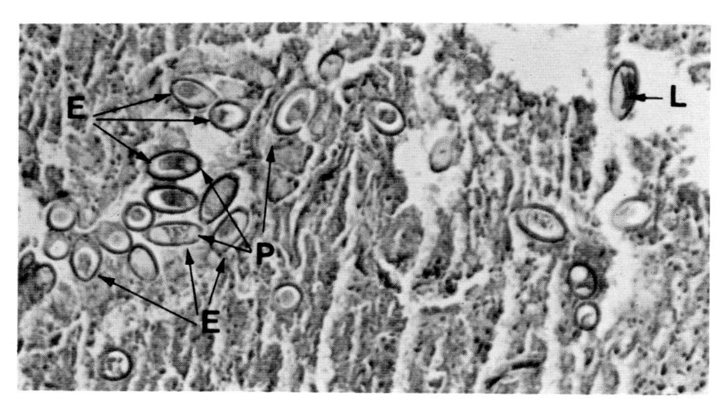

Fig. 12. Maggot of a fly in the appendix.
The cross section of a routinely sectioned appendix removed at an autopsy reveals a somewhat crushed maggot (M) of a fly. There is no apparent tissue reaction. The final diagnosis was made by the unsectioned half of the dipterous larva recovered from the appendix in which it had been stuck. (x12)

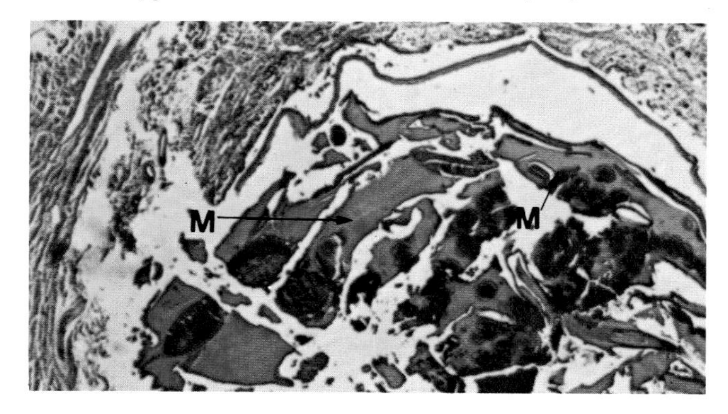

where larvae live until mature and ready for further development outside. Experimental intestinal myiasis seems to indicate that maggots of some species of flies, when swallowed, may survive the passage through the gastrointestinal tract of man but do not establish themselves for any length of time in the mucosa and are immediately evacuated. The possibility of accidentally being entrapped in the appendix, although remote, does exist.

Large tapeworms

The three large tapeworms of man, *Taenia solium* (pork tapeworm), *Taenia saginata* (beef tapeworm), and *Diphyllobothrium latum* (fish tapeworm), live in the small intestine. In spite of their large size (*T. solium* 2-4 meters, occasionally 8 meters in length; *T. saginata* 4-10 meters, occasionally 25 meters; *D. latum* 3-10 meters), the large tapeworms are seldom observed in their adult stage in tissue sections. Although rare cases of severe injury to the intestinal wall, including perforation are reported to be produced by *T. solium*, usually only slight, superficial irritation of the intestinal mucosa is found. This may be produced even by the unarmed scolex of *T. saginata*. The only time when a large tapeworm may be found in a tissue section is when a detached segment, the proglottid, is seen in the lumen of the appendix. The proglottids of *T. saginata* are found more often than those of other large tapeworms even in areas endemic of the latter two. The frequency with which the large terminal proglottid of the beef tapeworm, measuring 16-20/5-12mm., penetrates the narrow lumen of the appendix occurs because it usually detaches itself from the worm singly while a whole chain of terminal proglottids is separated from the pig tapeworm. The proglottids of *D. latum* disintegrate after egg laying within the intestine. The proglottid of *T. saginata*, once detached from the worm, is more active than the sluggishly moving segments of *T. solium*. Sometimes, even immature segments of *T. saginata* may be found in the appendix. This is probably due to early disintegration of a very long chain, aided by strong peristalsis. The role of *T. solium* in the tissues is important, not in its adult but in the larval stage, as cysticercosis. The larva of the pork tapeworm, the *Cysticercus cellulosae* may be found in tissue sections in numerous organs of man.

Ova of *T. saginata* may be found in a section of an appendix, often singly, but occasionally in a large mass. While the gravid proglottid of *T. solium* has to be crushed or digested in order to liberate its eggs, a proglottid of *T. saginata* easily releases its uterine contents of eggs through the anterior border after separation from the tapeworm. This explains

Fig. 13. Taenia saginata in the appendix.

Two proglottids (P) of *T. saginata* in cross-section. The segment of a tapeworm in a section may be recognized by its elongated form and undulating wall (W). These two proglottids are not gravid as there are no eggs within the central uterine cavity (UC). Although the mucosa of the appendix is not unusual, there is a little hemorrhagic inflammatory exudate (IE) between the appendicular mucosa and one of the proglottids, as well as between the two proglottids. (x12)

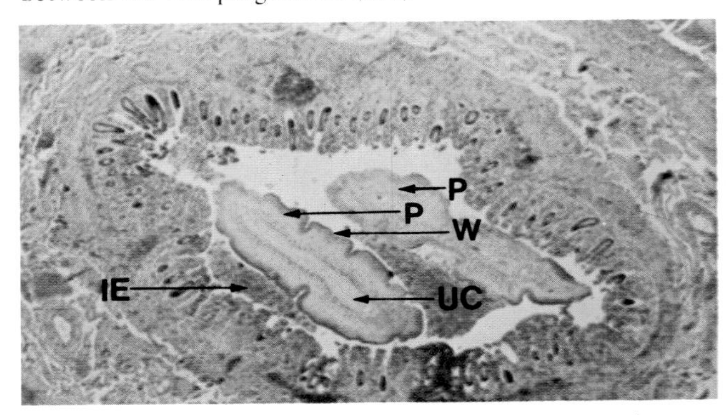

Fig. 14. Taenia saginata in the appendix.

In this section, part of *T. saginata* proglottid is examined at a high magnification. The proglottid (P) demonstrates the characteristic morphology of a tapeworm, with its smooth undulating cuticle (C) and loosely arranged, palisade-like wall of muscle cells (MC) beneath it. To the right of the proglottid, inflammatory exudate (IE) contains mononuclear cells, neutrophils and a few eosinophils. (x400)

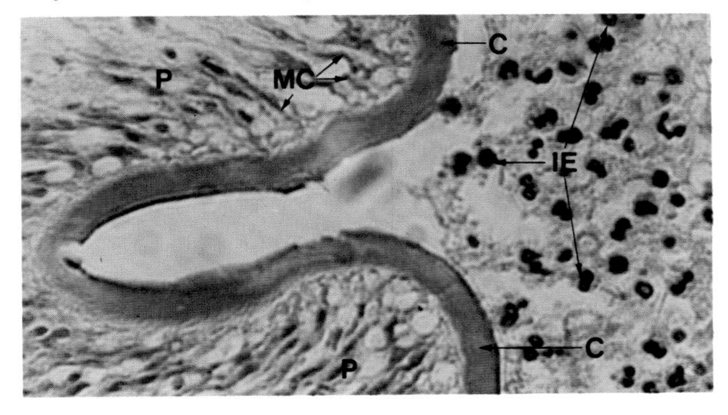

the massive expulsion of the eggs from a large gravid, active proglottid of *T. saginata* trapped in a narrow lumen of the appendix. The eggs of *T. solium* are practically never found in the appendix, which is gratifying to pathologists since there is no way of differentiating the eggs of *T. solium* from those of *T. saginata.* The eggs of both species are round or slightly elliptical, measuring 32-35 microns in diameter. When mature, the *Taenia* eggs contain a round, fully developed, light-brown embryo with six hooklets. These embryophores are recognizable by their thick covering membrane perforated by minute canals, giving the periphery of the eggs a striated appearance.

Small tapeworms

One of the small tapeworms of man *Echinicoccus granulosus* (Hydatid tapeworm), is of importance only in its larval stage when it produces the hydatid cyst. Two other accidental human infections with small tapeworms, *Dipylidium caninum* (the dog tapeworm) and *Hymenolepis diminuta* (the rat and mouse tapeworm), require an intermediate host for transmission. The intermediate hosts in which the larval stage occur are the dog flea, for *Dipylidium caninum,* and fleas, beetles and other insects for *Hymenolepis diminuta.* In order to acquire an infection with these two small tapeworms, man must swallow their intermediate hosts, which is not a frequent occurrence. Such infections do occur in children but these parasites are practically never found in tissue sections.

The third occasional small tapeworm of man, *Hymenolepis nana* (dwarf tapeworm) has a life cycle that makes the infection of man easier. This parasite does not require an intermediate host and man gets infected by swallowing food contaminated with the mice feces containing the infective eggs of the tapeworm. This is particularly true where mice population are not controlled. The gravid proglottid of *H. nana* easily disintegrates in the intestine of the mouse and the liberated eggs are fully infective when passed in the feces. The swallowed egg liberates a larva in man's intestine. The larva becomes attached to the mucosa of the small intestine and in 10-12 days develops into an adult parasite. After about 30 days the adult parasite produces infective eggs which appear in the feces of man with frequent reinfection and even autoinfection. Man, therefore, is the common host of *H. nana* and may harbor as many as 1,000 parasites. The adult *H. nana* is attached to the mucosa in the upper 2/3 of the ileum by means of a ring of 20 to 30 hooklets on a retractile rostellum, a protrusion on the scolex of the tapeworm. *H. nana* would be more frequently

Fig. 15. Ova of *Taenia saginata* in the appendix.
Numerous eggs (E) of *Taenia saginata* found in the lumen of a sectioned appendix. A similar picture would be observed within the uterus of a gravid proglottid of *Taenia* stuck in the appendix. The mature eggs are dark, and have a capsule (CAP) with a striated appearance. (x250)

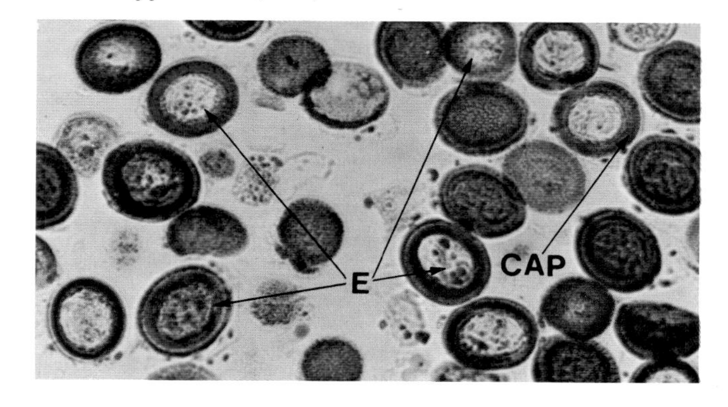

Fig. 16. Hymenolepis nana in the small intestine.
H. nana in a longitudinal section demonstrates a protruded rostellum (R) on its rounded scolex (S). The neck (N) of the tapeworm is almost as thick as the head and the proglottids (P). (x100)

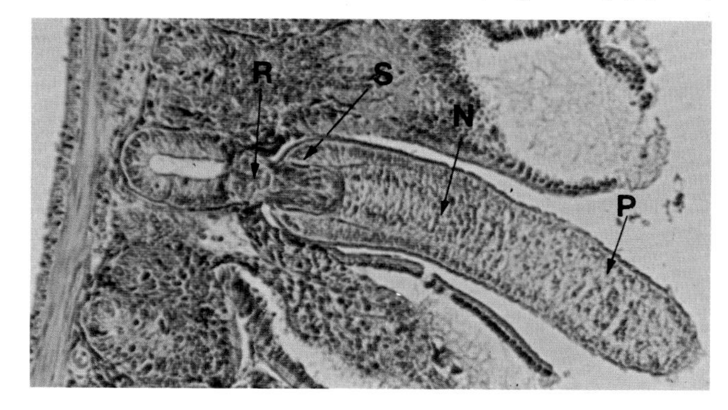

observed in tissue sections if it were not overlooked at autopsy because of the size of this small tapeworm, only 5-45/0.5-0.9mm. Although a heavy infestation may give rise to a severe general toxemia, local injury to the intestine results only in mild enteritis.

Strongyloides stercoralis

This small nematode is primarily a parasite of man. It has a complex life cycle comprising a direct cycle within the body of the host and a free living cycle outside the human body. The infection is acquired by active penetration through the skin of slender, infective filariform larvae of *Strongyloides.* Before developing into adult worms of the intestine these infective larvae, like those of the *Ascaris,* migrate through the right heart and lung of the man. In light infections, the adult *S. stercoralis* is usually restricted to the duodenum and upper jejunum. In heavy infections it is common to find the parasites throughout the whole length of the small and large intestine and even in the proximal biliary and pancreatic passages. The female worm measures 2.2/0.04mm. and is readily observed in the sections of the intestinal mucosa. The male worm, which is three times smaller than the female, is never found in tissue sections. Perhaps the male, unlike the female, does not penetrate the mucosa but is eliminated soon after copulation which takes place in the lumen of the intestinal tract. The female deposits only a few eggs at a time. These thin-shelled, transparent eggs, measuring 50-58/30-34 microns, are well segmented when deposited by the female after fertilization. The eggs hatch small noninfective rhabditiform larvae which are eliminated with the feces and are either transformed into infective filariform larvae or start the free living cycle outside the body. A section of the intestine may reveal adult females of *S. stercoralis,* well segmented eggs, and more numerous larvae.

The only other larvae of nematode worms which may be found in the mucosa of the small intestine are those of *Trichinella spiralis.* The differential diagnosis between the two is not difficult. The larvae of *S. stercoralis,* 225/16 microns, hatch out of the eggs which are deposited superficially in the intestinal mucosa. The smaller larvae of *T. spiralis,* 80-120/5.6 microns are deposited in the deepest layers of the mucosa. Since the female of *T. spiralis* is viviparous and never deposits eggs but releases larvae, no eggs can be found in trichinosis. The larvae of *S. stercoralis* must reach the lumen of the intestine to complete their life cycle while those of *T. spiralis* must reach the deep lymphatics and the bloodstream to complete theirs. Thus, it is use-

Fig. 17. Strongyloides stercoralis in the small intestine.

The longitudinal section of the small intestine demonstrates numerous round larvae of *S. stercoralis.* The larvae (L) are cut either longitudinally or across but the details are undistinguishable at this magnification. However, one can observe that some are escaping into the lumen of the intestine, which is characteristic for the rhabditiform, noninfective larvae of this species. (x35)

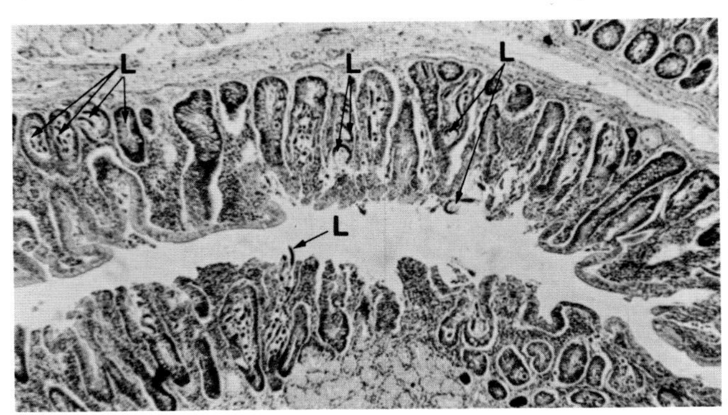

Fig. 18. Strongyloides stercoralis.

Small rhabditiform larvae (L) of *S. stercoralis* in the mucosa of the small intestine are mostly sectioned across but occasionally are sectioned lengthwise. The larger structures, center, are eggs (E) of *Strongyloides.* These differ from cross-sections of the female worms by their obvious segmentation in morular stage which gives the egg an uneven, mulberry-like contour. (x100)

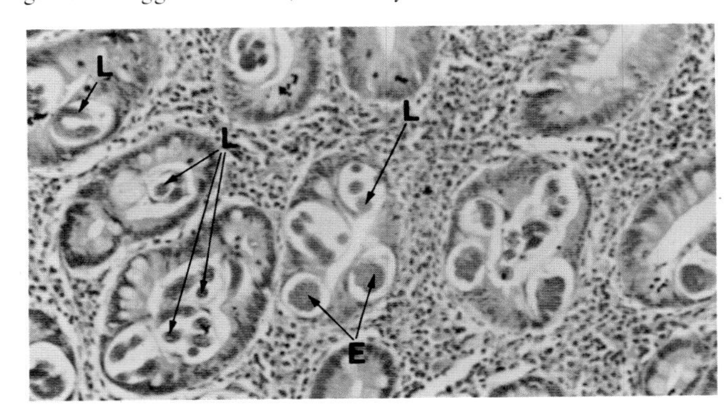

Fig. 19. Ova of *Strongyloides stercoralis* in the small intestine.

Two well segmented eggs of *S. stercoralis* in the mucosa. Note the thin, practically invisible capsule (CAP) and the very transparent quality of the eggs outside the central cellular division (CCD). (x400)

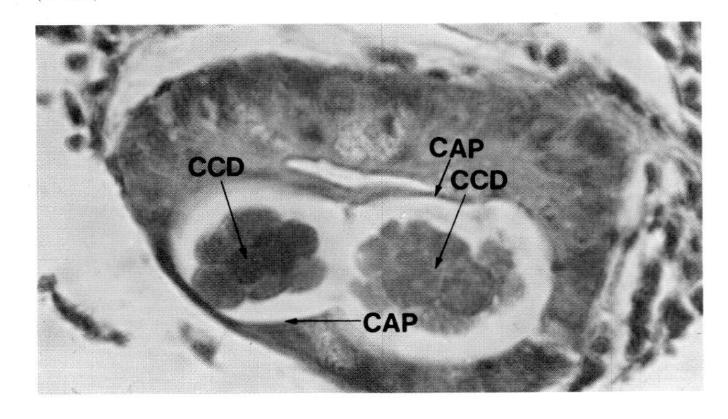

ful to study longitudinal sections of the small intestine to observe the larvae of *Strongyloides* emerging into the lumen.

Hookworms

Human species of hookworms, *Necator americanus* (the New World hookworm), originally brought to the United States from West Africa, and *Ancylostoma duodenale* (the Old World hookworm) are seldom found in tissue sections even in hyperendemic areas. Yet, people harboring these parasites are estimated to number over 700 million throughout the world, with these parasites constantly attached to the intestinal mucosa because they are blood feeders. Human infections with *Ancylostoma braziliense*, a parasite of dogs and cats, have also been reported in man. The human species of hookworms are small, cylindrical, off-white nematodes, measuring 5-13/0.3-0.6mm., the variation being related to species and sex. The species, which can be easily identified in wet mounts by differences in the structure of their buccal cavities and genital organs, can hardly be recognized in tissue sections. Unlike many species of parasites, the proportion of male and female hookworms is about equal. The posterior extremity of the male is considerably broader than the rest of the parasite. It is formed by a bursa, a membranous structure containing finger-like rays, with which the male parasite holds the female during copulation. The hookworm's normal location in the host is the upper part of the small intestine but in heavy infections it can be found the whole length of the small intestine. The main criterion for recognizing a hookworm, in a tissue cross section, is the relatively thick cuticle, and its wide open mouth sucking the mucosa which is apparent in both cross and longitudinal sections. A longitudinal section passing through the posterior end of the parasite showing the presence of the bursa helps to differentiate a male hookworm. As with *S. stercoralis*, hookworm infection in man occurs through the skin usually between the toes and the back of the feet. Infective filariform larvae can be found in skin sections during the time of active penetration of the skin. Just as in *Strongyloides* and *Ascaris*, the cycle within the human host includes migration of the filariform larvae through lymphatics and veins to the right heart and lungs before reaching its final destination in the small intestine.

Macracanthorhynchus hirudinaceus

This worm is an accidental parasite of man. Its natural hosts are hogs, wild boars and accidentally dogs and cats. However, it is a cosmopolitan parasite and its rarity in man can be ascribed to the fact

Fig. 20. Hookworm in the small intestine.
A longitudinal section of a male hookworm (H) demonstrates the open mouth (M) holding the intestinal mucosa (IM), left, and the wide candal bursa (B) to the right. (x35)

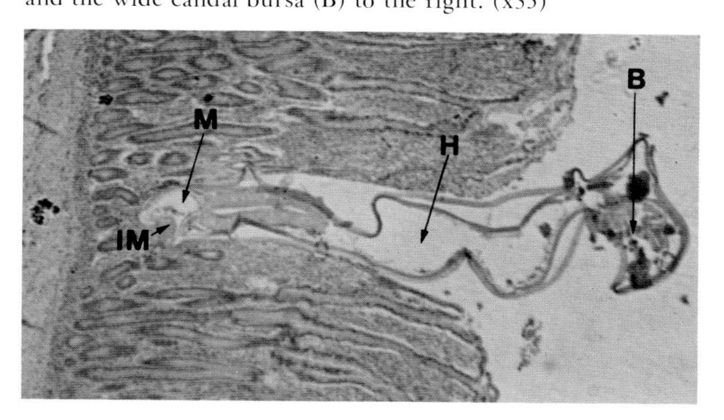

Fig. 21. Hookworms in the small intestine.
The cross-section of a hookworm (H), right, demonstrates the internal structures and the characteristic thick outside cuticle (C). Left, a lengthwise section of another hookworm shows the open mouth (M) buried deep in the mucosa. To the right of the mouth is the contractile well developed esophagus (E) with which the parasite sucks the blood from its host. (x40)

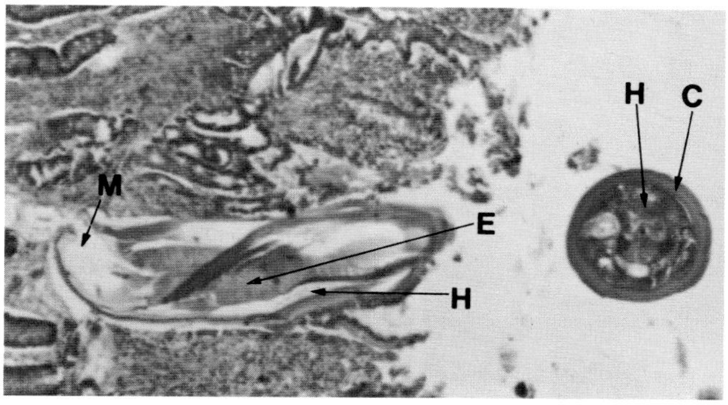

Fig. 22. Hookworm in the small intestine.
A cross-section of the head of a hookworm (HW) showing the characteristically wide open mouth (M) with intestinal mucosa (IM) pulled into it. (x100)

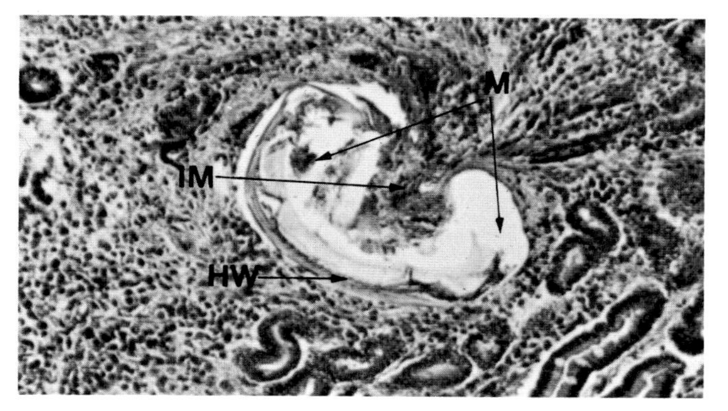

that its life cycle includes an intermediate host, a beetle which must be swallowed to acquire the infection. Perhaps the short life span of *M. hirudinaceus*, one year or less, limits the spread of the infection among men. The parasite is a milky-white worm, measuring 5-65cm./3-10mm. It has a peculiar, wrinkled appearance, and a retractile proboscis on its rounded anterior end which is armed with 5 or 6 rows of spines. The parasite is attached to the mucosa of the intestine, and the resultant damage to the intestinal wall ranges from localized inflammation to severe hemorrhagic necrosis which may result in an intestinal perforation.

Capillaria philippinensis

The natural reservoir of this parasite is unknown. Although man appears to be only an accidental host, thousands of human cases have been reported during the last few years. It has been suggested that this unusual frequency may be related to the particular raw fish diet of the local population in the Philippine Islands. Laboratory animals, such as monkeys and wild rats, have been experimentally infected with larvae of *C. philippinensis* found in species of fresh water fish. The eggs of *C. philippinensis* resemble those of *T. trichiura* except that they are slightly smaller, their polar structures are flatter, and their shells slightly pitted. Because the eggs contain a fully developed larva when released by the female, the possibility of autoinfection appears very plausible.

These small nematodes measure 2.3-4.3mm./3-47 microns. The female is larger than the male and both are attenuated toward the ends. A cross-section of *C. philippinensis* varies greatly depending on where the parasite is sectioned. The anterior portion which in the female is half of the total length but is shorter in the male contains the esophagus and esophageal glands. The posterior portion is occupied by the reproductive system and the intestines. The parasites are imbedded in the mucosa of both the small and large intestine. If untreated, they may cause a severe inflammatory reaction resulting in intractable diarrhea, emaciation and death.

Schistosomes (blood flukes)

The three most important trematodes of man—blood flukes, are more commonly found than any other parasite in tissue sections. All three species of human schistosomes, *Schistosoma mansoni*, *Schistosoma japonicum*, and *Schistosoma haematobium*, are wide spread in vast areas of the world, depending upon the presence of suitable snail intermediate hosts and poor sanitary conditions. The animal reservoir of natural hosts is impressive. A large

Fig. 23. Macracanthorhynchus hirudinaceus.
A cross-section of the anterior end of *M. hirudinaceus* (M.h.) within a hemorrhagic area (HA) of severely damaged wall of the small intestine demonstrates the characteristic, externally situated spines (S). (x12)

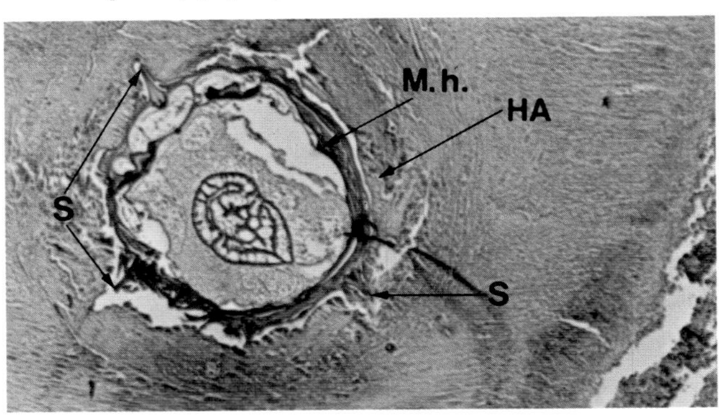

Fig. 24. Macracanthorhynchus hirudinaceus.
The anterior end of *M. hirudinaceus* (M.h.) in longitudinal sections, penetrating a hemorrhagic necrotic intestinal wall. The anterior spines (S) in this section are not as apparent as in the cross-section but the characteristic rugose appearance (RA) of the parasite is well demonstrated. (x12)

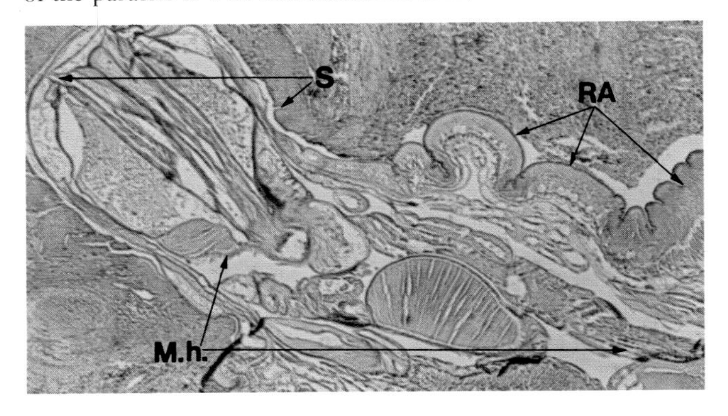

Fig. 25. Capillaria philippinensis in the small intestine.
Both the cross-section (CX) and the oblique section (OX) of the anterior extremity of *C. philippinensis* are visible. There is a marked infiltration of the mucosa by mononuclear cells and an occasional eosinophil on the left. (I) is small intestine. (x400)

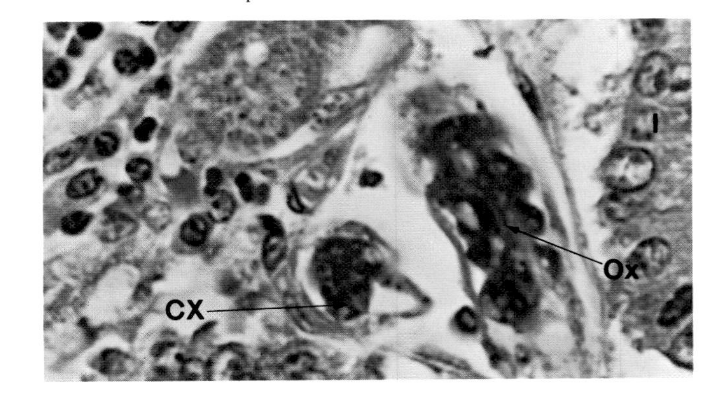

Fig. 26. Ovum of *Schistosoma mansoni* in pressed rectal mucosa.

The egg (E) of *S. mansoni*, in a longitudinal position demonstrates the diagnostic lateral spine (S). There is a somewhat deformed miracidium (Mi) in the egg. Unstained. (x100)

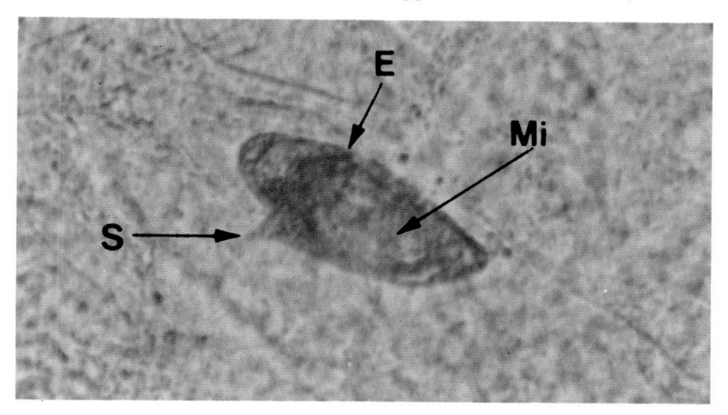

Fig. 27. Ova of *Schistosoma mansoni* in the intestinal submucosa.

Many longitudinally sectioned eggs of *S. mansoni* are visible. The egg on the right clearly demonstrates the characteristic lateral spine (S), and a well-stained miracidium (Mi). (x100)

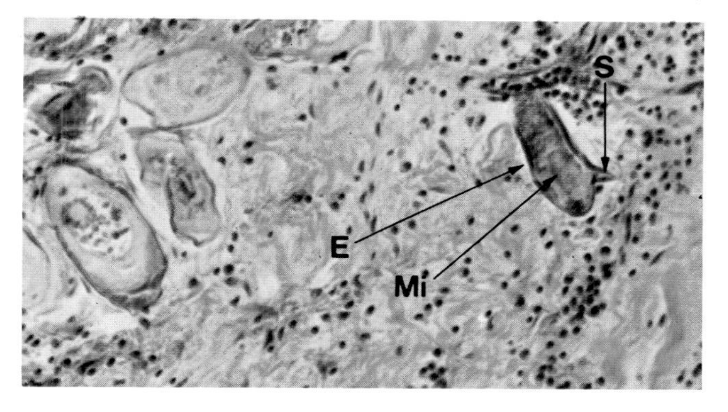

Fig. 28. Ova of *Schistosoma mansoni* in mesenteric venules.

Two eggs (E) of *S. mansoni* are sectioned longitudinally and one crosswise in small venules of the mesorectum. The egg to the far right shows the unmistakably diagnostic lateral spine (S) as does the cross-sectioned egg. All three eggs contain miracidia (Mi) pointing to an active schistosomiasis. (x100)

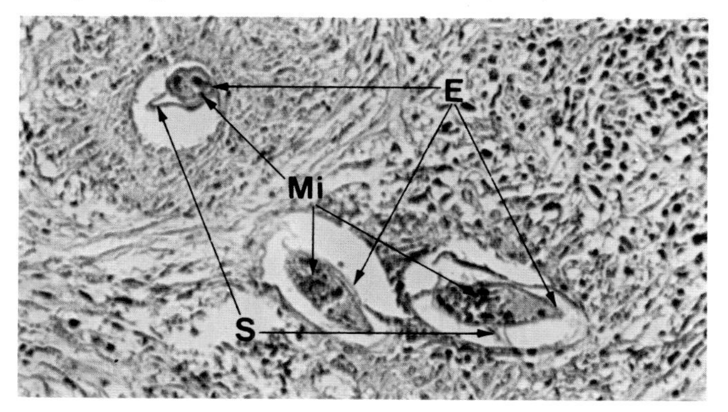

number of animals not normally found to carry schistosomiasis have shown experimentally to be suitable to harbor these parasites. The adult worms are estimated to have a longevity of up to 30 years. According to their maturity and species, schistosomes live in the portal, mesenteric or vesical venous circulation. The eggs, which are normally eliminated through feces or urine may also be widely disseminated throughout the body and found in tissue sections of practically any organ.

The adult schistosomes, particularly the males, have a characteristic appearance and are easily recognizable. They measure, from the smallest, *S. mansoni*, to the largest, *S. japonicum*, 10-26/0.3-0.56mm. The males are shorter, stouter, and have a ventrad infolding forming the gynecophoric canal. This canal is open all the way from the ventral sucker in front to the posterior end of the parasite. The slender and longer female is held in this canal during copulation. There seems to be a much closer relationship between the two sexes of schistosomes than of many other parasites. In fact, the presence of the male is necessary for the maturation of the adolescent female, and once together, the male and female seldom separate. Thus, couples are often linked together when time for oviposition of the gravid female has arrived. Perhaps this extended duration of copulation may somehow be responsible for the greater dissemination of the aberrant eggs. The slim, long body of the female is physiologically adapted to reach deeply into small venules to lay one egg after another, slowly withdrawing to fill the narrow venule with eggs. Under pressure and using the spines and lytic enzymes, the eggs leave the venule to escape into the intestine or the urinary bladder, according to their species. The eggs are eliminated with the feces or urine, and the life cycles of the schistosomes are completed outside the body. When laying the eggs while still being embraced in the gynecophoric canal of the shorter but wider male, the female cannot reach far into the very narrow venules. It is obvious that the eggs laid in a larger venous channel, under less pressure and lesser contact with the venous endothelium, may be more easily swept away by the bloodstream. Stranded eggs of *S. mansoni* and *S. japonicum*, laid in venules around the intestines would naturally be swept toward the portal circulation, and the majority would be filtered out by the liver. Others may go through or by-pass the liver and be found in the gallbladder, pancreas, stomach, lungs, and even the central nervous system. The female of *S. japonicum* because of its larger size cannot penetrate the smallest venules. Its more numerous smaller eggs do not have a true spine to

Fig. 29. Ova of *Schistosoma japonicum* in the mesentery.

The numerous eggs (E) of schistosomes in this section all appear to be sectioned crosswise. The diagnosis of *S. japonicum* and not of *S. mansoni* should be considered in spite of some of the eggs exhibiting spine-like (SL) processes. These "spines" are multiple in many eggs indicating that they actually are cracked eggshells. Furthermore, not a single one of these eggs is the size to suggest an egg of *S. mansoni* sectioned lengthwise. Longitudinal sectioning would inevitably occur with so many eggs present if they belonged to *S. mansoni* species. (x40)

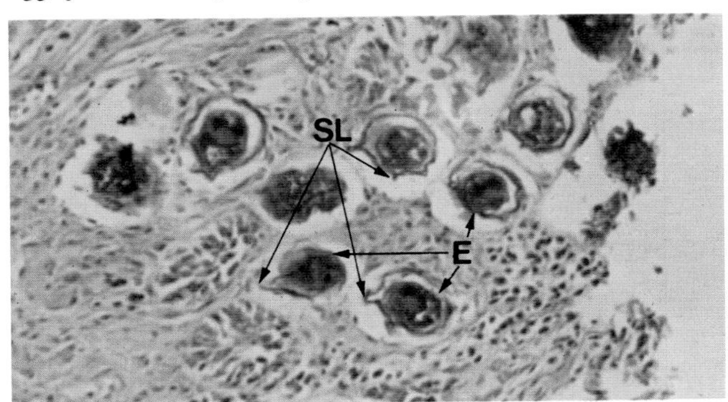

Fig. 30. Adult *Schistosoma mansoni* in the mesentery.

There are two males (♂) and three females (♀) of *S. mansoni*. All of the schistosomes are present as cross-sections. (x40)

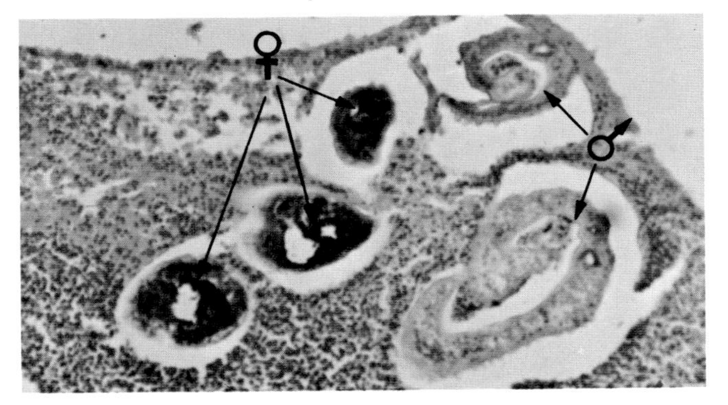

Fig. 31. Adult *Schistosoma mansoni* in a mesenteric vein.

One *S. mansoni* male (♂) holding a female (♀) in his gynecophoric canal (GC) during copulation. The female is sectioned obliquely and therefore, appears longer than the two cross-sectioned females in the same small mesenteric vein. (x40)

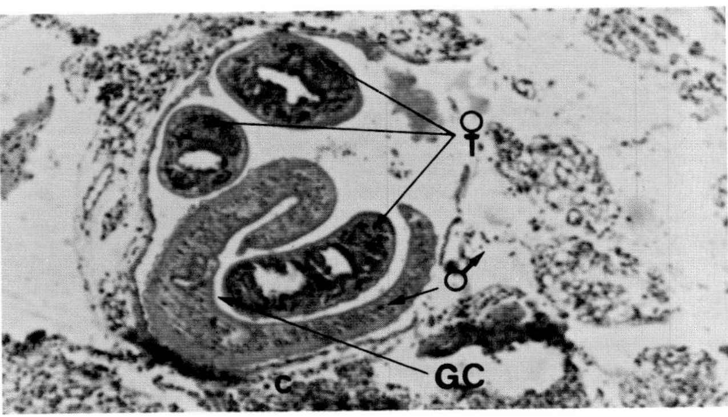

Fig. 32. Adults of *Schistosoma mansoni.*

There are two couples of *S. mansoni* during copulation, both sectioned longitudinally, in mesenteric veins. The female (♀) (left) in the gynecophoric canal of the male (♂) is coiled which makes it appear to be in multiple sections. The female (right) within the male over the lymph node (LN) is straight. (x12)

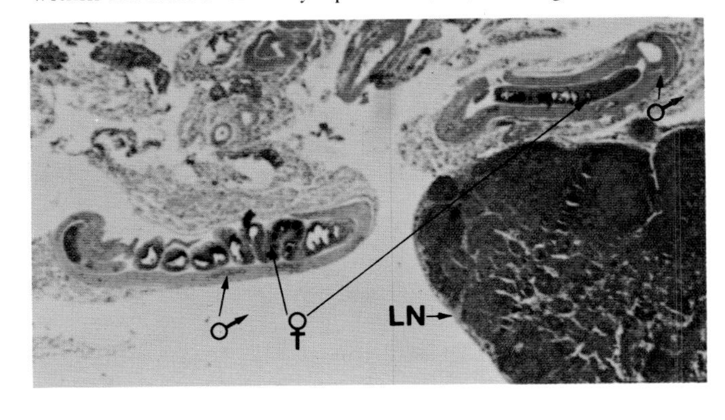

Fig. 33. External cuticle of the male *Schistosoma mansoni.*

The integument of a cross-sectioned male (♂) *S. mansoni*, high magnification, demonstrates the characteristic prominent but unevenly high, rounded tuberculations (T), which are diagnostic of this species. (x400)

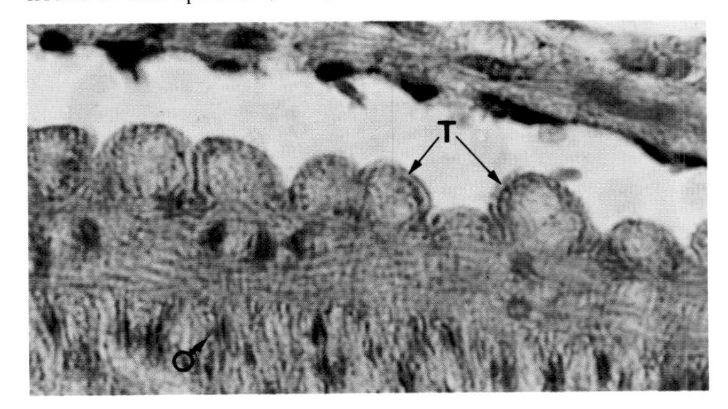

initiate the penetration of the endothelium. Therefore, the eggs of this species of schistosome are more likely to be swept away by the bloodstream than those of the other two species. The great majority of the eggs deposited by *S. haematobium* are found in the submucosa of the urinary bladder. However, many may be found in adjoining organs or if carried along by the bloodstream may be found in distant locations. Eggs of *S. haematobium* have been found in the uterus, kidney, vagina, ovaries, spleen, and organs even more distant from the bladder.

As with other parasites, the differentiation of species is more difficult in tissue sections than in wet mounts of the parasites. Diagnostic criteria such as the point of reunion of the two bifurcated ceca, number of testes, or number of eggs within the gravid female, aiding in establishing the species of a whole parasite, are not practical in tissue sections. Only occasionally may diagnostic morphological criteria be observed in sections, e.g., the integument of *S. mansoni* is strongly tuberculated, much less conspicuous in *S. haematobium*, and completely smooth in *S. japonicum*.

The eggs of *S. mansoni*, measuring 114-175/45-68 microns, and those of *S. haematobium*, measuring 112-170/40-70 microns, are easy to recognize in longitudinal sections because of their spines which are lateral in the former and terminal in the latter. It is more difficult to identify the smaller, more elliptic eggs of *S. japonicum*, 70-100/50-65 microns. The lateral spine of this egg is minute and rarely detectable even in wet mounts.

Sometimes the long, pointed lateral spine of a *S. mansoni* egg in a cross section is quite visible and appears as a single spine on a well rounded egg. If there appears to be more than one lateral spine in a cross-section of an egg, it probably is not a spine but the result of a cracked egg shell and the differential morphological diagnosis between *S. mansoni* and *S. japonicum* is virtually impossible. When there are numerous round or oval eggs all appearing in cross-section they are probably eggs of *S. japonicum*, even if they occasionally appear to have spines. In fact, the rule of averages suggests the likelihood that an occasional egg among many will be sectioned longitudinally revealing its greater length and perhaps, the true spine, should they belong to *S. mansoni* species.

It is important to observe in a tissue section whether an egg contains a miracidium, a ciliated larval form. This form within an egg indicates the presence of live, active, mature schistosomes, whereas its absence may indicate an old, inactive infection.

The cercariae, the infective stage of the schistosomes, released from infected snails are practically never found in skin sections because this invasion period is very short and the tissue response is minimal. The developmental forms of schistosomes are seldom found during their migration from the skin, via the bloodstream, through the right heart and lungs. Their presence in the lungs, unlike that of the infective larvae of *Ascaris*, is very brief, although tissue reaction to the adolescent schistosomes may sometimes result in pneumonitis.

The adult worms usually do not elicit any severe tissue reaction during their sojourn within the venous system. However, the dead worms traveling with the venous current toward the portal circulation, may produce severe inflammatory reaction within the vein that results in thrombosis and may lead to fibrosis of the vessel wall.

It is the eggs of the schistosomes, beginning with their forceful passage out of the venules, and following their deposit in various tissues, that produce the real tissue damage. This damage may range from minute pseudotubercles and small granulomas with only a few eggs deposited in the tissue to severe and extensive changes of the invaded organ when the eggs are numerous. In the intestinal wall, constant infiltration by eggs may lead to extensive fibrosis resulting in late complications such as adhesions, constrictions, hemorrhages, etc. In the urinary bladder, extensive irritation and damage to the submucosa may culminate in carcinomas. Numerous aberrant embolic eggs may produce extensive changes even in distant organs, e.g., severe cirrhosis of the liver or right ventricular failure of the heart due to repeated injury to the lungs. Sometimes a few embolic eggs may even be the cause of disastrous results when they lodge in strategic areas of the brain.

Hydatid cyst (Echinococcus granulosus)

The normal host of the adult *E. granulosus* is the dog to which the parasite became adapted from its original hosts, wild carnivorous animals. The most important intermediate host which carries the hydatid cyst is the sheep. After swallowing an egg of *E. granulosus* which may be deposited on anything soiled by feces of an infected dog, man harbors the larval stage, i.e., the hydatid cyst, as the intermediate host. The frequency with which man contracts the dreaded hydatid cyst is related to the geographical distribution of *E. granulosus*. The frequency is increased in sheep-raising countries and with man's close association with infected dogs. The embryo of *Echinococcus*, after liberating itself from the ingested egg, makes its way through the intestinal wall into the mesenteric circulation and may either start its development in the mesentery or is carried to any part of the body, even the bones. Most often the hydatid cyst is found in the liver.

Hydatid cysts may be unilocular or when derived from *Echinococcus multilocularis,* alveolar. The unilocular cyst, the common variety, is usually single and grows slowly. It is made of an anuclear, laminated wall surrounded by fibrous reaction of the invaded tissue and an internal thin, nucleated germinal membrane. Attached to the latter and bathing in a pale-yellow fluid are daughter cysts, identical to the original cyst. The germinal layer also produces brood capsules which contain scolices armed with hooklets. When swallowed, a scolex develops into an adult *E. granulosus* in the intestine of the new host, thus completing the life cycle. Actually, the brood capsules are often detached and broken within the cyst, liberating the scolices into the hydatid fluid and are then called "hydatid sand." A well preserved hydatid cyst with its germinal layer intact and the daughter cysts, brood capsules and scolices still attached to the germinal layer is seldom observed in tissue sections. Even if removed unruptured from an organ the cyst is often traumatized during laboratory processing. It is often necessary to search within the section for scolices or their hooklets, the latter being found singly or in crown formation. The difficulty of finding hooklets is increased in old calcified cysts or in alveolar cysts of *E. multilocularis* which seldom produces scolices in man. The best technique to aid in locating the hooklets is to use the acid fast stain. When the cyst is sterile no scolices or hooklets can be found and the diagnosis has to be made on the basis of the external, characteristically laminated, anuclear cyst wall.

When an active hydatid cyst ruptures within the body, the secondary metastatic cysts are established by dissemination. Cysts often spread to the immediate proximity, e.g., from the liver to the peritoneal cavity or to the lung. However, they may also reach distant locations like the eye or the brain. The pathogenesis and the tissue reaction depend upon the exact location of the cyst. The size depends largely upon the space available for expansion of the slowly growing cyst which may occasionally reach up to 20 cm. The morbidity is also related to the pressure effect from the expanding cyst. Conversely, silent asymptomatic cysts have been known to exist up to 30 years.

Fig. 34. Hydatid cyst of *Echinococcus granulosus* in the mesentery.

Part of an old hydatid cyst of *E. granulosus* is examined at a low magnification. From the left upper corner to the right lower corner one can see the following: remnants of a thin, nucleated germinal layer (GL) of the cyst, darkly stained; anuclear, laminated cyst-wall (CW) containing colorless spaces of cholesterol crystals (CC); fibrous reactive tissue (FT) of the mesentery; adipose (AT) and lymphoid (LT) tissue. A.F. (x50)

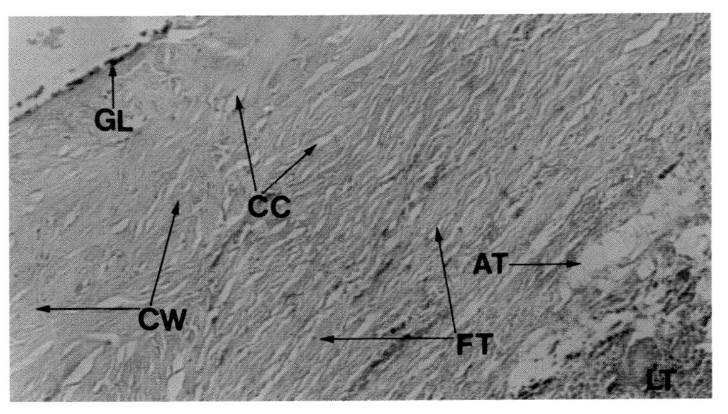

Fig. 35. Scolices of *Echinococcus granulosus* within a hydatid cyst.

Five well preserved scolices (S) of *E. granulosus* are presented in the longitudinal or oblique sections. One can see crowns of hooklets (CH) within the scolices. (x100)

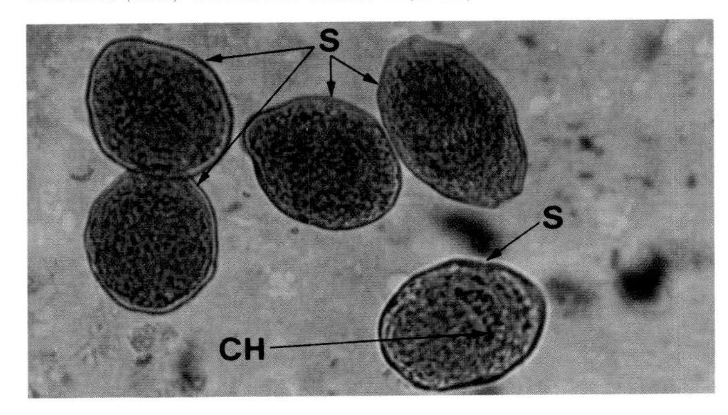

Fig. 36. Hooklets of *Echinococcus granulosus* in an old mesenteric hydatid cyst.

Numerous diagnostic hooklets (H) of *E. granulosus* in the hydatid sand (HS) are stained dark red with the selective acid fast stain. In addition to the hooklets with their characteristic form there are also parts of hooklets. These parts and hooklets are from scolices completely disintegrated in this old hydatid cyst. A.F. (x250)

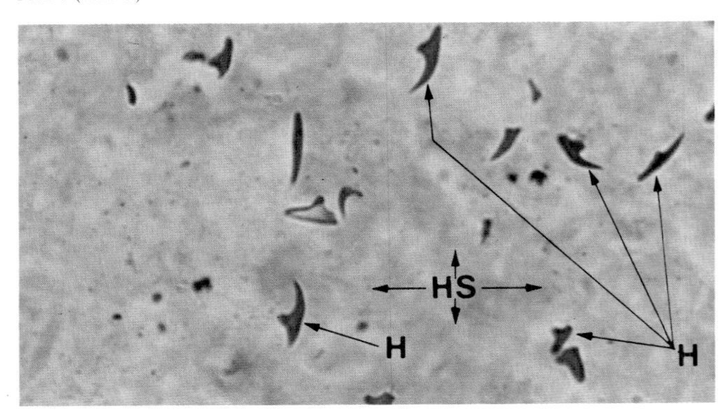

Liver

Like any other organ, the liver is the predilection site of parasites adapted to live in its environment, e.g., *Fasciola hepatica*, the liver fluke. Because of its strategic location between the portal venous system and the general circulation, the liver serves as a giant trap for many parasites or their eggs, e.g., eggs of schistosomes swept away by the blood current from the venules in which they were deposited. Futhermore, organisms which use reticulo-endothelial cells for symbiotic parasitism, as in visceral leishmaniasis, find an ideal site in the Kupffer cells of the liver. Thus, the tissue sections of this large organ may reveal a number of parasites, some expected, others purely accidental.

Fig. 37. Ovum of *Schistosoma mansoni.*
The egg (E) of *S. mansoni*, sectioned longitudinally, is in a granuloma (G) of the liver. The lateral spine of the egg is not visible in this section. The egg contains a miracidium (Mi) testifying to the presence of adults of both sexes within the host. Among the cells surrounding the egg are many lymphocytes and plasma cells and also some eosinophiles. (x250)

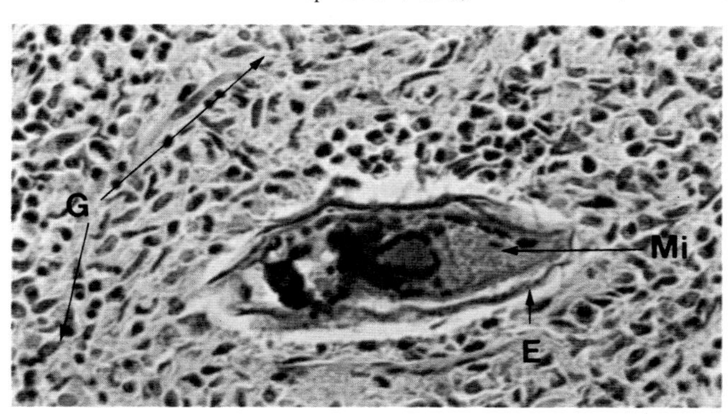

Fig. 38. Ovum of *Schistosoma mansoni* in the liver.
The egg (E) of *S. mansoni* is cross-sectioned. None of the visible outside protrusions represent the lateral spine but merely evidence of shrinkage and cracking of the eggshell. There is a miracidium (Mi) within the egg. Around the egg there is a granulomatous tissue reaction. (x250)

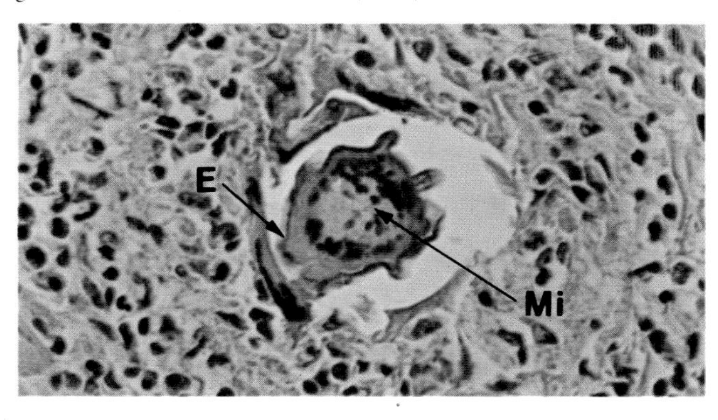

Fig. 39. Two ova of *Schistosoma japonicum* in the liver.

The two cross-sectioned eggs (E) of *S. japonicum* look identical with the egg of *S. mansoni* in Fig. 38, except that they are stained with a special stain. Therefore, the positive diagnosis on one or two eggs in such a cross-section without a clearly visible lateral spine of *S. mansoni* is not possible. The blue area of fibrosis (F) around the two eggs, made discernable by the special stain, shows the extent of the tissue reaction in the liver. Both eggs contain miracidia (Mi). Trichrome. (x100)

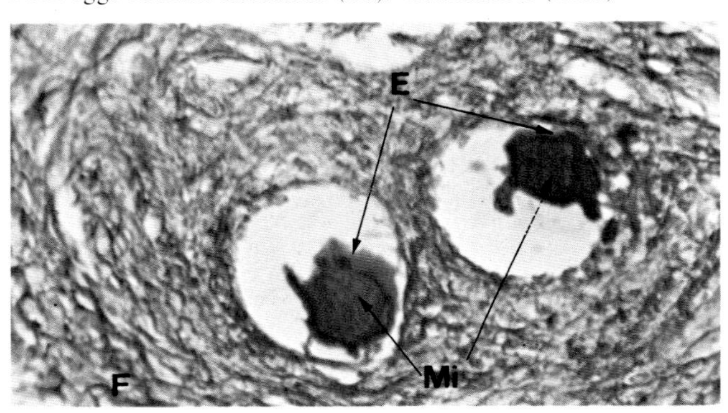

Fig. 40. Calcified adult worms of *Schistosoma mansoni* in a portal vein of the liver.

Two calcified adult *S. mansoni* (S.m.) must represent dead worms swept by the blood current from mesenteric veins. The diagnosis was confirmed by the medical history of the patient and by numerous eggs of this species found in the liver. The portal vein (PV) shows evidence of thrombosis (T). The normal architecture of the tissue around the vein is obliterated. (x40)

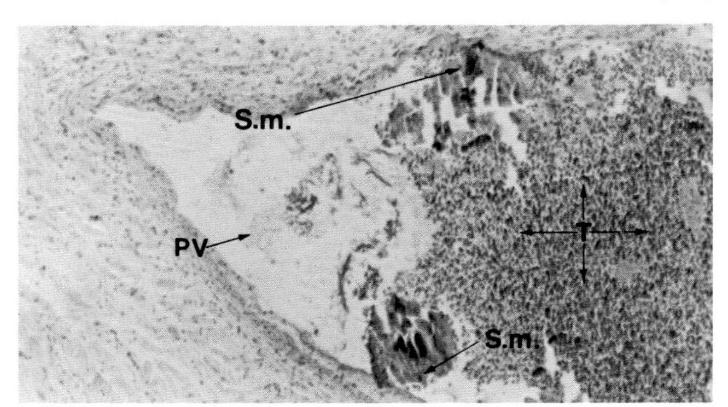

Fig. 41. Leishmania donovani.

The reticulo-endothelial cell (REC) is filled with *Leishmania* (L) organisms in an overwhelming infection. In spite of this massive invasion of the cell, there is an impression that the parasites do not tend to form a compact aggregation like a cystic structure. Near practically every nucleus (N) of *Leishmania donovani* there is a kinetoplast (K) in either linear or pinpoint form. The nucleus of the host cell is to the right. There are a few *Leishmania* outside the cell. Giemsa. (x1,000)

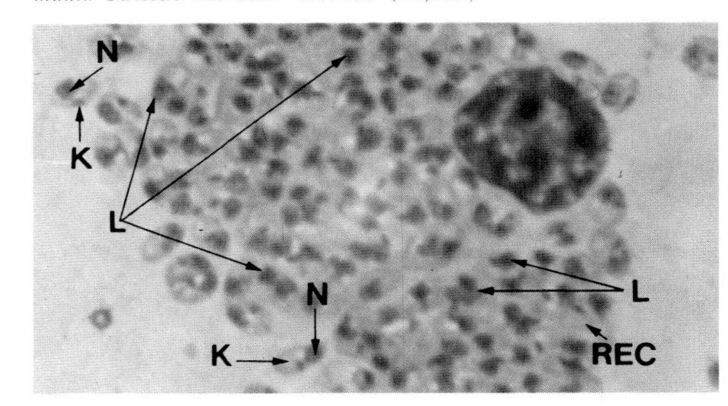

Fig. 42. Leishmania donovani.

Kupffer cells in a liver section contain numerous *L. donovani* (L.d.). The diagnostic kinetoplasts are not clearly demonstrable but the loose arrangement of *Leishmania* in the macrophages is characteristic. There is a marked proliferation of Kupffer cells (KC) bordering the dilated sinusoids. (x1,000)

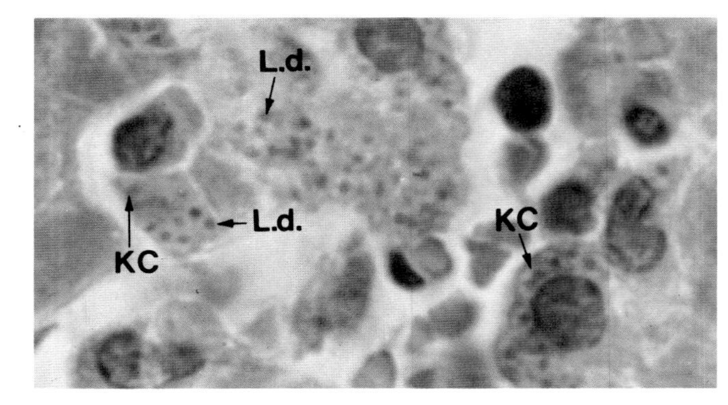

Leishmania

Leishmaniasis is a disease caused by a protozoan organism. Man is the main host of this parasite which exists on all continents except Australia. The *Leishmania* genus contains three species affecting man: *Leishmania donovani*, (causing visceral leishmaniasis, kala-azar, dumdum fever, black disease), *Leishmania braziliensis*, (American leishmaniasis, mucocutaneous leishmaniasis), and *Leishmania tropica*, (Oriental sore, cutaneous leishmaniasis). All three are usually transmitted by various species of *Phlebotomus*, the sand fly. In visceral form, transmission has also been reported through blood transfusions and even through coitus. *L. donovani* apparently has multiple strains prevalent in certain areas and varying in their host reservoir and response to treatment. The *Leishmania* of all three species is morphologically identical. A typical *Leishmania* is an oval protozoan, measuring 2-4/1-3 microns. Its main diagnostic feature is the presence of a rod-shaped kinetoplast near its rounded nucleus. While the kinetoplast is seen in practically every parasite on a stained smear or tissue imprint, this minute structure seldom appears in tissue sections. In order to establish an absolute diagnosis, the kinetoplast must be found. *Leishmania* is an intracellular organism which uses symbiotic parasitism to multiply and spread within the infected organ. Therefore, it is usually found in reticulo-endothelial cells of the organ, e.g., the Kupffer cells of the liver, or the blood macrophages, which may be present in any organ. While visceral leishmaniasis affects mainly the spleen, the liver, the lymph nodes and the bone marrow, it can be found in many other organs of the body, including the skin. The cutaneous leishmaniasis attacks the skin only and the mucocutaneous species only mucous membranes and the skin. The basic pathologic lesion of each organ invaded by *Leishmania*, is the enormous multiplication of the cells in which this parasite thrives. Thus, the liver is enlarged due to excessive proliferation of Kupffer cells. However, the organisms may also be found in macrophages derived from the blood.

In the liver *L. donovani* must be differentiated from *Toxoplasma gondii*. The latter does not have the kinetoplast near the nucleus as seen in *Leishmania*. Therefore, kinetoplasts provide the diagnosis when they are present in the section. The kinetoplast may appear either as a rod-like structure or as a pinpoint body located near the nucleus. Even if it cannot be demonstrated with the certainty under oil immersion, an impression that not all nuclei are of the same size, may indicate that the small structures may be kinetoplasts. Furthermore, while *Leishmania* organisms tend to be loosely spread over the host cell, the *Toxoplasma* tend to be packed together to form a cystic formation. Contrary to *Leishmania* this cystic structure does not fill the whole parasitized cell, leaving the periphery free of parasites.

Toxoplasma gondii

Toxoplasmosis is a cosmopolitan infection with a high rate of incidence but a relatively low percentage of symptomatic disease. It may be either congenital or acquired. In the latter, it is more pathogenic during the early, acute stages after which it may become dormant or inactive. Although the exact mode of transmission is not known, there are indications that toxoplasmosis is contracted through ingestion of contaminated food, such as meat and eggs. In feline hosts the infective stage has proved to be a resistant coccidian oocyst. However, the only form of *Toxoplasma* which has been found in tissue sections in man is the trophozoite in the invaded organ. It is a pyriform protozoon measuring 4-7/2-4 microns with an oval nucleus situated closer to the rounded posterior extremity of the parasite but it contains no kinetoplast. *T. gondii* has a predilection for nervous tissue such as retina and brain but may be found in viscera and muscles. When located in sections of the liver and heart it has to be differentiated from *Leishmania*, whereas in skeletal muscles *Sarcocystis lindemani* must be ruled out. In acute infections *T. gondii* may be found singly or in small groups while in chronic infections it is usually observed in cysts without a capsule. Sometimes, when it spreads to the neighboring cells, *Toxoplasma* tends to continue to form compact cyst-like groups, smaller and smaller in size, giving the formation a tadpole appearance.

Fig. 43. Toxoplasma gondii.

The cyst (C) of *T. gondii* in the liver does not fill the whole cell but leaves the borders of the cell free. There is no definite limiting cyst capsule, except perhaps, for a slight host cell tissue reaction. The nuclei (N) of the *Toxoplasma* organisms are all about the same size. (x1,000)

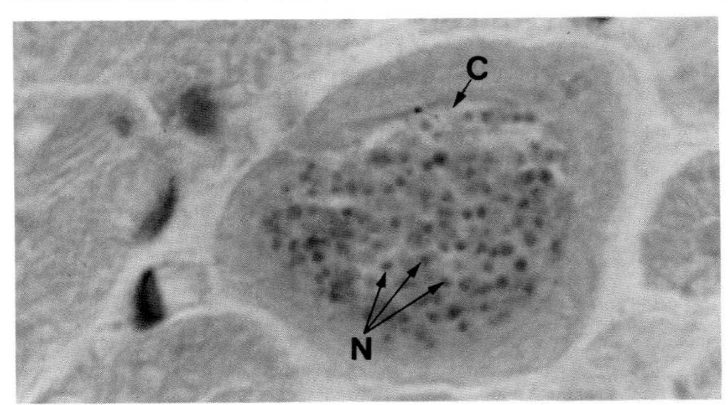

Fasciola hepatica

This large, flat cosmopolitan fluke, measuring 2-3/0.8-1.3cm., is the parasite of herbivorous animals. It requires a snail as an intermediate host to complete its life cycle. Man usually acquires the infection by eating plants like watercress infected with metacercariae, the encysted cercariae released from the snail. The adult parasite is usually located in a bile duct of the liver where it may be found in tissue sections. However, the larval stages of *F. hepatica*, after being swallowed and having perforated the duodenal wall to migrate to the liver via the lymphatics and veins, may get lost. Such aberrant parasites occasionally wander into other organs where they may be discovered.

The pathology of *F. hepatica* infection ranges from early eosinophilic infiltration and encapsulation of the parasite to obliteration of bilary passages and liver cirrhosis, the latter enhanced by the deposition of eggs, 130-150/63-90 microns, within the liver tissue. The diagnosis of *F. hepatica* in tissue sections can be made by the large size of the fluke and by the presence of multiple sections of small intestinal diverticula within the parasite. These diverticula are small branches of two divergent ceca running the whole length of the parasite and are diagnostic features of this species. Occasionally, the diagnosis may be made by finding the eggs in the tissue section of the organ.

Fig. 44. Fasciola hepatica.

A cross-section of *F. hepatica* (F.h.) and a part of a second one in a bile duct (BD) of the liver. The size of the parasite and its characteristic form are sufficient to differentiate it from another frequent invader of the bile duct, the *Clonorchis sinensis*. The presence of multiple branches of the ceca (BC), appearing as small ducts lined with glandular cells, are diagnostic of the species. There is some deposit between the parasite and the bile duct due to desquamation of the biliary epithelium. (x12)

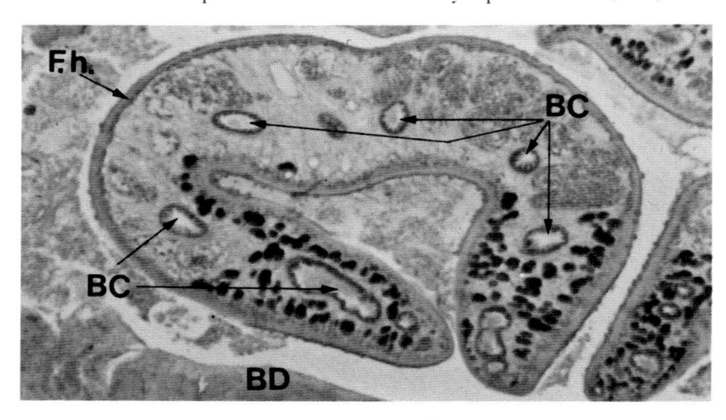

Clonorchis sinensis

The oriental liver fluke, a parasite of man and fish-eating mammals, is restricted to the Far East. Infections have been reported in other countries, e.g., Hawaii, where the suitable snail, the first intermediate host, does not exist. This has been explained by ingestion of raw, infected fish imported from endemic areas. The adult parasite inhabits the bile ducts of the host. Although it is a small trematode measuring only 12-21/2.8-5.0mm. with great variations within these dimensions, the pathologic changes caused by clonorchiasis may be very severe, depending on the number of flukes. In slight infections the parasites move around in the biliary passages and the changes may be limited to simple eosinophilic infiltration and slight thickening of the walls of the duct. However, in heavy infections, sometimes by thousands of flukes, there is progressive periductal fibrosis, cirrhosis of the liver, and often secondary bacterial infection leading to biliary obstruction and other severe complications. The diagnostic criteria used to recognize the whole parasite, such as its attenuated, elongated form, characteristic posterior, deeply lobed testes, one in front of the other, etc., seldom help in tissue sections. How-

Fig. 45. Clonorchis sinensis.

The section of the bile duct (BD) of the liver contains many *C. sinensis* (C.s.) cut at various angles. Some flukes contain numerous eggs (E) in sections of the coiled uteri. On the periphery, the bile duct shows some thickening and the liver is compressed. (x12)

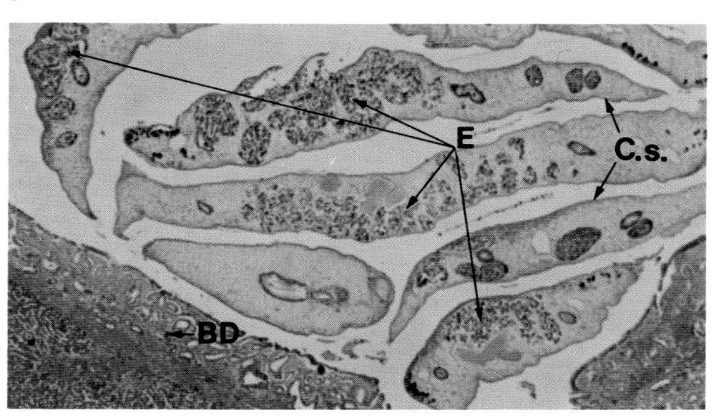

ever, the long closely coiled and convoluted uterus, often full of eggs, is frequently found in sections and does help the diagnosis. When a single *C. sinensis* is found sectioned crosswise, without the uterus in the section, the measurement is important. A careful examination with a higher magnification will often reveal characteristic eggs between the parasite and the biliary duct. These eggs measure only 27-35/12-20 microns, their shape is often compared to the old-fashioned electric light bulb, with the operculum situated at the narrower anterior end and clearly visible. This operculum rests on a thickened end of the eggshell, as on small shoulders. The posterior end of the egg has a button-like thickened protuberance.

Capillaria hepatica

Although primarily a parasite of rats and other rodents, animals such as dogs, cats, wild pigs, monkeys, and occasionally man can be infected. The adult parasites resemble *T. trichiura*, but unlike the latter which live in the large intestine they invade the parenchyma of the liver. The eggs deposited by the female in the liver do not mature and cannot be eliminated. In order to complete the life cycle of *C. hepatica* these eggs must be ingested together with the infected liver by another carnivorous animal. The eggs pass undamaged through the intestinal tract, are eliminated in the feces, mature, and must be swallowed to finally form adult parasites in the liver of a new host. Only occasionally do eggs deposited in the liver find their way through

Fig. 46. Clonorchis sinensis in a bile duct of the liver.
Part of a *Clonorchis sinensis* (C.s.) at a high magnification reveals within the uterus of the parasite, numerous sections of eggs and each contains a darkly stained miracidium (Mi). The special stain demonstrates the extensive fibrosis (F) of the liver beyond the bile duct (BD) and some connective tissue within the duct itself. Trichrome (Masson). (x40)

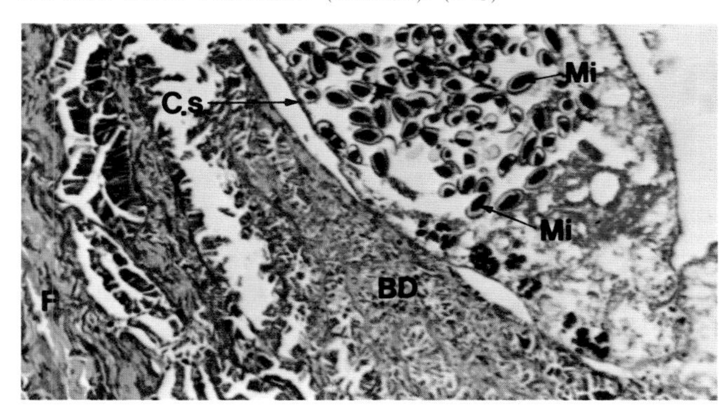

Fig. 48. Ovum of *Clonorchis sinensis.*
An egg (E) of *C. sinensis*, between the integument (Int) of the fluke to the right, and the epithelium of the bile duct (BD) to the left, reveals its characteristic elongated form, slightly narrowing toward the anterior end, a miracidium (Mi) inside, and the thin, yellow-brown shell (S) with the small operculum (OP) fitted into the thickened rim of the "shoulders" (Sh). (x400)

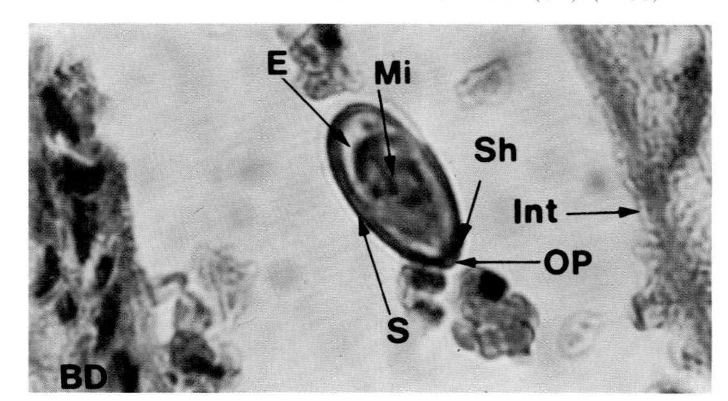

Fig. 47. Clonorchis sinensis in the bile duct of the liver.
Part of a single *C. sinensis* (C.s.) in cross-section shows the typical thin external cuticle (C), the loose structure of its stroma, and the anterior sucker (AS). Between the fluke and the bile duct (BD) are a few eggs (E) which assist in the diagnosis. (x40)

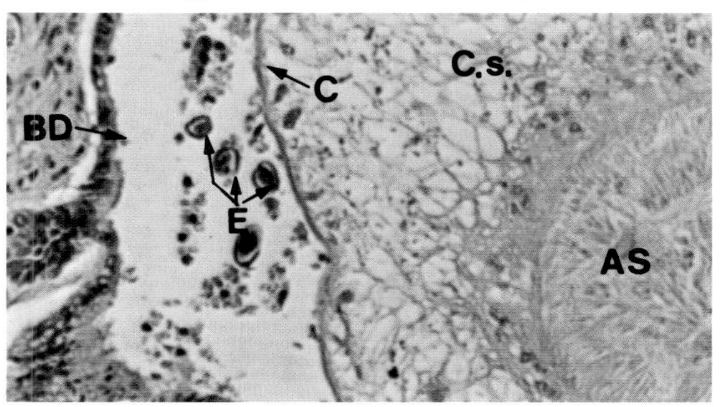

Fig. 49. Capillaria hepatica in the liver.
The cross-section of an adult *C. hepatica* (C.h.) and its eggs (E) are surrounded by intense granulomatous reaction (IGR) in the liver tissue. (x250)

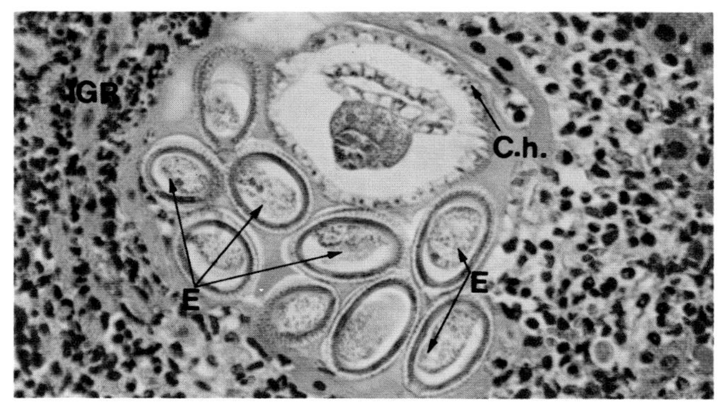

Fig. 50. Capillaria hepatica eggs in the liver.

Two eggs (E) of *C. hepatica* sectioned at different angles reveal their characteristic, diagnostic features. These eggs are very similar in form to those of *T. trichiura*. However, the eggshell (ES) is not smooth, but pitted, and appears beaded. The terminal plug-like (P) structures are not rounded and do not protrude outside the eggshell. (x540)

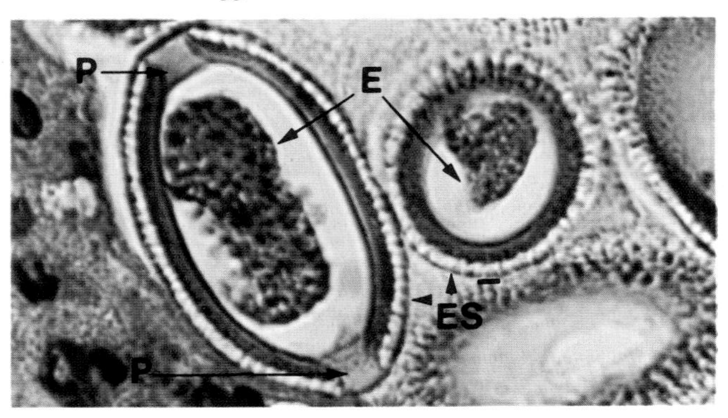

Fig. 51. Visceral larva migrans in the liver.

The cross-sectioned small visceral larva migrans (L) shows under its integument, the typical long muscle fibers (MF) which are characteristic of the *Ascaris* species. To the left, there is a multinucleated foreign body giant cell (GC) frequently found in tissue sections with visceral larva migrans. (x400)

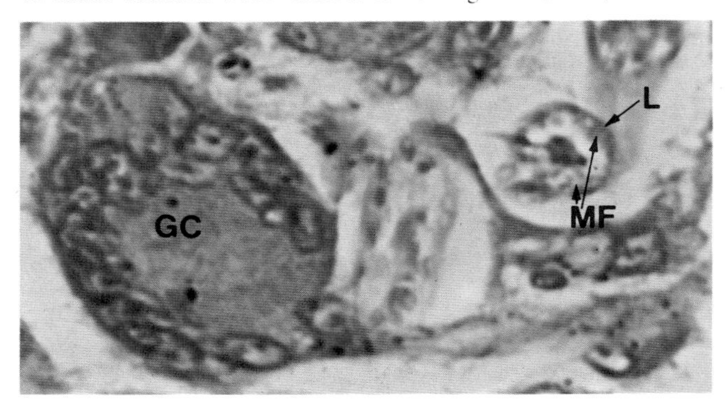

Fig. 52. Ascariasis in the liver.

This is a cross-section of an *Ascaris* egg (A) within an abscess formation. The mammillated coating (MC) is preserved on all sides of the embryonated egg. Such an egg in the liver parenchyma suggests that an *Ascaris* has invaded a bile duct. (x400)

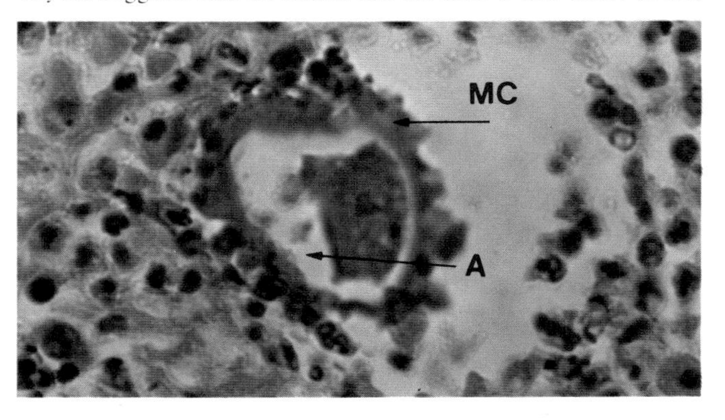

the biliary ducts into the intestine and are present in stool examination of an infected man. Finding the typical eggs of *C. hepatica* in the feces of man does not necessarily mean that his liver is infected but may indicate the consumption of the liver of an infected animal. Usually the diagnosis of capillariasis in man is made on tissue sections after an autopsy and more rarely on liver biopsy. Since the life span of the adult parasites is very brief the diagnosis in the liver sections can be made while the characteristic and very resistent eggs remain present. They resemble the lemon-shaped eggs of *T. trichiura* but are slightly larger, up to 68 microns in length, their outer shells are very characteristically pitted and in sections appear beaded or segmented. The terminal plug-like structures of the eggs appear to stick out less than those of *T. trichiura*.

A liver infected with *C. hepatica* may demonstrate all degrees of damage, from mild early hepatitis to late necrotic changes and cirrhosis.

Visceral larva migrans

This is a condition resulting from the invasion of man's organs by larval stages of nematodes which are unable to complete their normal life cycle. The most common cause of visceral larva migrans in man is an infection resulting from swallowing a mature egg of *Toxocara canis*, the dog's *Ascaris*, or of *Toxocara cati*, the cat's *Ascaris*. The normal life cycle of these parasites in their natural hosts is similar to that of *Ascaris lumbricoides* in man. This cycle includes a migration of the larva, liberated from the swallowed egg, from the small intestine to the right heart and lung, then to the bronchioles and the trachea, again swallowed, to finally reach the small intestine for the second time and develop into an adult parasite. When man swallows an egg of *T. canis* or *T. cati*, the larva liberated in the man's intestine tries to complete its usual life cycle. But once in the bloodstream of man, it is lost in the unfamiliar physiological surroundings of an unknown host. It may wander for weeks, sometimes for months, before getting entrapped in the capillaries of an organ where the larva finally dies. The damage to the organ where the larva is located depends on the location, the tissue reaction, and the sensitivity of the host, enhanced by repeated infections. The usual tissue reaction is an eosinophilic granuloma but in a hypersensitive host a focal necrosis is often observed. Visceral larva migrans has been found in a number of organs, such as the liver, brain, eye, and other locations. It is often missed and tissue reaction may be attributed to other pathological conditions.

Sometimes, larvae of *A. lumbricoides* and hookworm larvae may become aberrant during their normal migration in man and such ectopic larvae produce a somewhat similar, although less severe reaction in the organ in which they had been trapped.

Furthermore, noninfective, rhabditiform larvae of *S. stercoralis*, which normally are eliminated with the feces of man and become infective filariform larvae outside the body, may sometimes undergo this change within the host. In such a case, the infective larvae act as if they had infected man through the skin and attempt to complete their life cycle by migrating via the bloodstream through the heart and lung. Among the many larvae involved in such an auto-infection some become ectopic visceral larva migrans.

Hydatid Cyst

Fig. 53. Hydatid cyst.
Part of a hydatid cyst in the liver (L) demonstrates its characteristic laminated capsule (LC). No germinative layer is visible but within the cyst there are numerous scolices (S) of *E. granulosus.* The liver parenchyma is compressed. (x40)

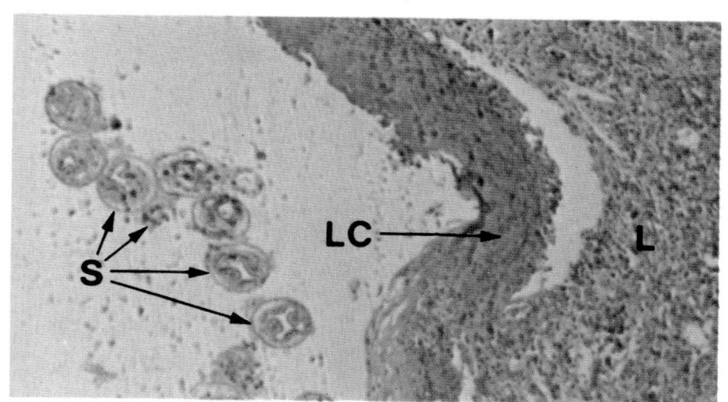

Fig. 54. Hydatid sand in an old hydatid cyst.
There are three oval structures that must represent old scolices (S) of *E. granulosus*, containing numerous rounded and oval calcified bodies, within an old hydatid cyst in the liver. Around the scolices are numerous colorless hooklets (H), singly or still in crowns. (x400)

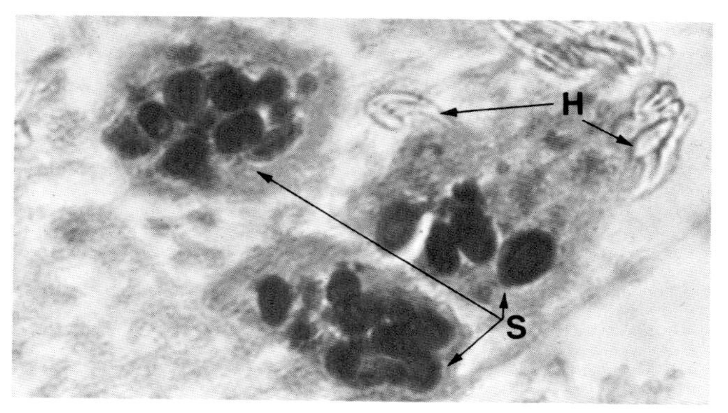

Fig. 55. Hydatid sand in an old hydatid cyst.
The dried-up, cracked hydatid fluid within an old cyst in the liver contains numerous crowns of hooklets (H) but no scolices of *E. granulosus.* (x100)

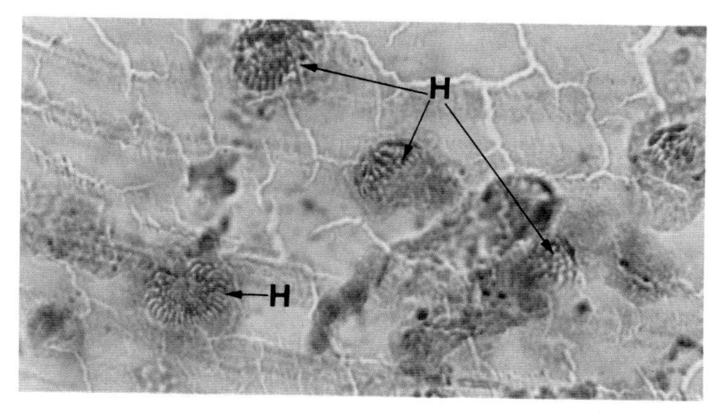

Fig. 56. Calcified hydatid cyst.
Part of an old calcified hydatid cyst in the liver demonstrates its thick, laminated capsule (LC) and two hooklets (H) of *E. granulosus*, fused together. The cystic cavity (CC) is completely calcified. (x540)

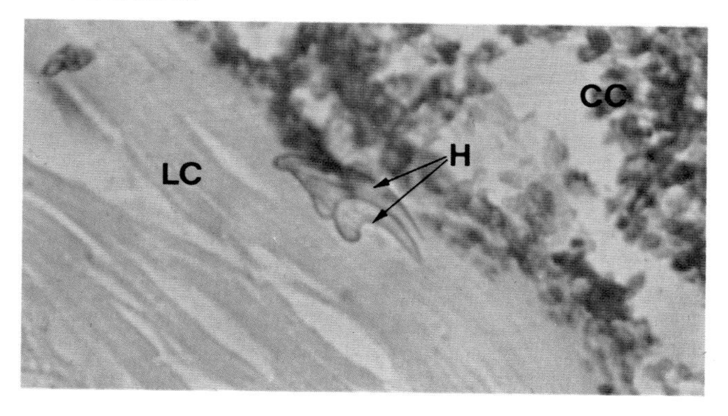

Fig. 57. Cyst of *Echinococcus multilocularis.*
A cyst of *E. multilocularis* in the liver demonstrates its characteristic septa (Sep), dividing the cystic cavity into multiple compartments, producing an alveolar type of cyst. Within the cyst are numerous brood capsules (BC) containing typical scolices (S). (x40)

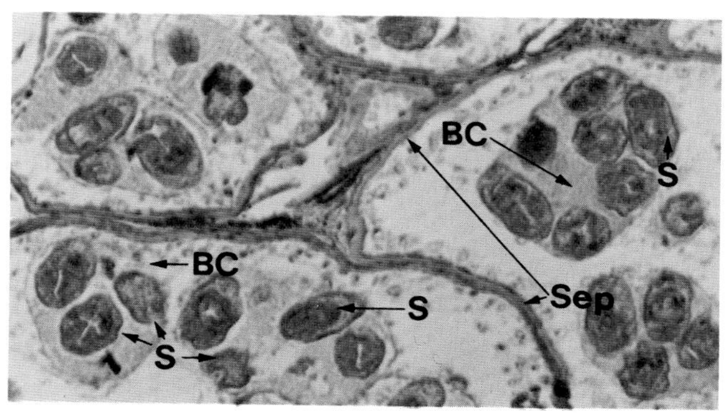

Malaria

Malaria of man involves four species of parasites: *Plasmodium falciparum, Plasmodium vivax, Plasmodium malariae,* and *Plasmodium ovale.* These protozoa are primarily parasites of the vascular system and are not found as easily in tissue sections as in peripheral blood smears. However, tissue sections reveal certain stages of malarial parasites that cannot be observed in the blood smears. When the sporozoites, the infective forms of malaria, are transmitted to man by a mosquito bite, these slender, spindle-shaped organisms 11-14 microns in length, find their way into the liver. They then initiate the pre-erythrocytic stage of the exo-erythrocytic cycle, so called because it occurs before the erythrocytes are infected. During this stage (which is not repeated in *P. falciparum* infections) the parasites actively multiply by asexual schizogony within the liver cells, resulting in the formation of 15,000 to 40,000 merozoites. These are parasites ready to enter the erythrocytes in which they will grow, multiply, and infect new erythrocytes during a repetitive erythrocytic cycle. Thus, the exo-erythrocytic stage may be observed in liver sections. This stage may occur more than once in species other than *P. falciparum.* Regardless, the diagnosis of malignant tertian malaria, due to *P. falciparum* in organ sections, is relatively easier than in malaria due to the other three species. *P. falciparum,* differing from the other three species, does not divide in the peripheral blood during the schizogony of the erythrocytic cycle but after some growth the parasites leave the peripheral blood and their division is accomplished within the capillaries of the organs. The number of parasites of *P. falciparum* are often greater than in other species of malaria. This results in a higher rate of erythrocytic destruction, a greater deposit of malarial pigment within the organs, greater hyperplasia of the reticuloendothelial system and other macrophages, more pronounced anoxia of those tissues not receiving enough oxygenated blood, and frequent obliteration of the capillaries by masses of dividing parasites. The conspicuous banana-shaped form of gametocytes, the pre-sexual forms of *P. falciparum,* is easier to recognize within the capillaries than the rounded forms of the other three species. Because of the remarkable regenerative capacity of the liver the usual pathological changes due to malaria, such as hyperplasia of the reticuloendothelial system, congestion, cloudy swelling or fatty infiltration, are neither spectacular nor characteristic except for the excessive accumulation of the dark malarial pigment, hemozoin. This is usually found in Kupffer cells but may be seen free in the capillaries. It is accompanied by a lighter colored hemosiderin, the pigment derived from hemoglobin released from the destroyed erythrocytes which is deposited in the parenchymal liver cells. The deposits of malarial pigment are easier to see than it is to find the malarial parasites. The massive pigment deposit in all organs in *P. falciparum* infections with frequent blocking of capillaries are characteristic enough to make the diagnosis of malignant tertian malaria even when examining a tissue section under low magnification.

Fig. 58. Pigment of *Plasmodium falciparum.*
A typical picture of hemozoin (H), the dark malarial pigment, deposited in the capillaries and accumulated within the Kupffer cells of the liver due to *P. falciparum* infection. (x1,000)

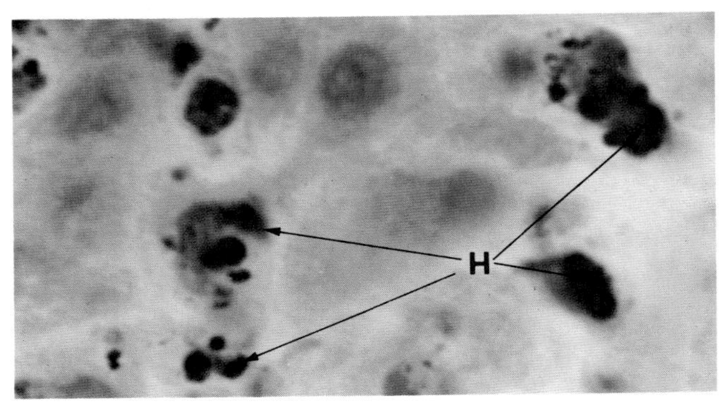

Fig. 59. Exo-erythrocytic cycle of malaria in the liver.
A highly magnified section demonstrates malarial parasites at the end of the exo-erythrocytic stage. The rounded, slightly irregular mass of dividing protozoa (DP) has formations of darker areas containing almost mature merozoites, ready to be released and invade the erythrocytes. (x1,000)

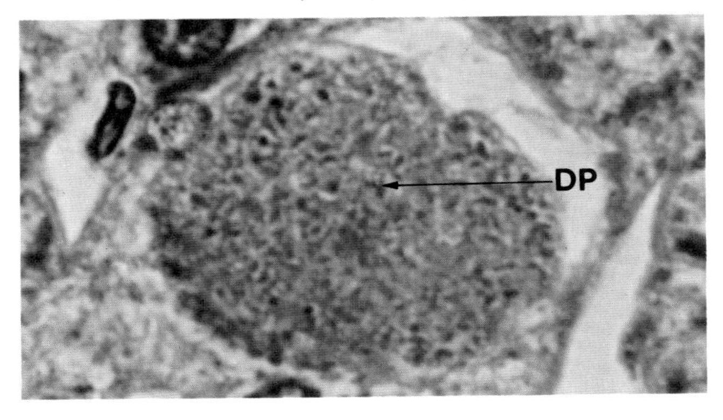

Spleen

The two most frequently found parasites in spleen sections are visceral leishmaniasis and malaria. This is probably due to the ease with which the reticuloendothelial system in the spleen responds to these two infections. The patterns of these two infections are similar to those that occur in the liver.

Fig. 60. *Leishmania donovani* in the spleen.
A marked hyperplasia of the reticuloendothelial cells of the spleen invaded by *L. donovani* (L.d.). In spite of an overwhelming systemic infection, the usual pattern of loose, uncrowded distribution within the macrophages is preserved. (x1,000)

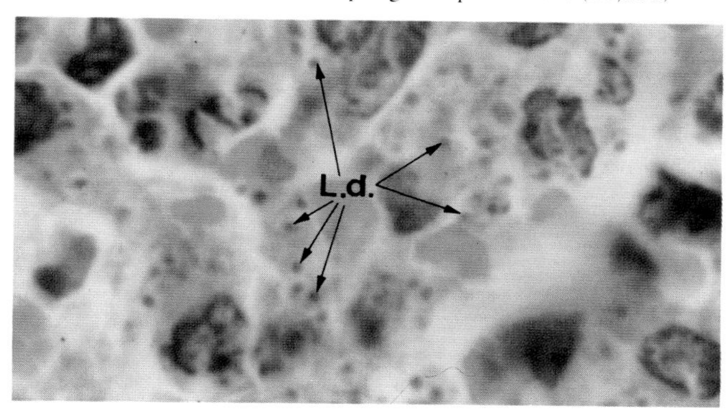

Fig. 61. Malarial pigment in the spleen.
The typical dark malarial pigment, hemozoin, concentrated within the capillaries and the phagocytic cells is seen throughout the spleen. (x400)

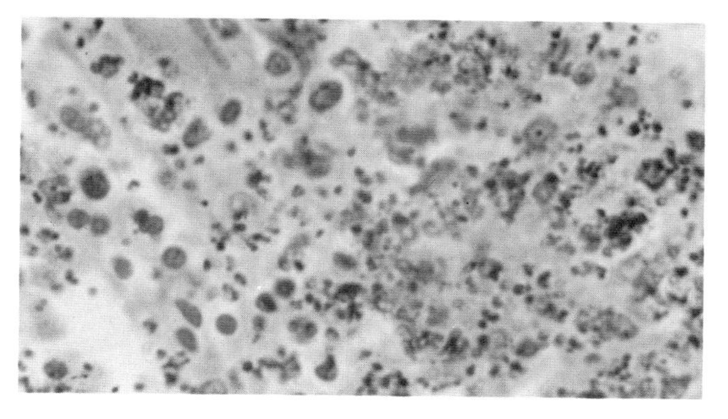

Stomach

Many parasites pass through the stomach of man in their life cycle. Some are parasites of animals or plants accidentally swallowed by man which are eliminated through the digestive system, e.g., coccidia of fish, or eggs of *Meloidogene marioni,* nematodes of the roots of plants. Others, parasites of man are harbored in the intestines and go through the stomach while completing their normal life cycle. Some of them pass through the stomach twice, e.g., *Ascaris,* once as an infective ovum after being swallowed and the second time as a young adolescent after having migrated through the heart and lung and being swallowed again. None of them affect the stomach and are rarely found in tissue sections. Some animal parasites, such as *Gnathostoma spinigerum,* or *Gongylonema pulchrum,* which normally encyst in the wall of the stomach are so rare as accidental human parasites that they do not pose a problem to either clinicians or pathologists. In summary, the only parasite which may be expected to invade the stomach of man and to be found in stomach sections are the aberrant eggs of schistosomes. This usually occurs in old infections concommitant with cirrhosis of the liver and an established collateral venous circulation through the gastric vessels.

Fig. 62. Ova of *Schistosoma mansoni.*
Three eggs (E) of *S. mansoni* in the mucosa of the stomach are visible. All three eggs contain miracidia (Mi). There is evidence of mononuclear cellular infiltration within the mucosa. (x100)

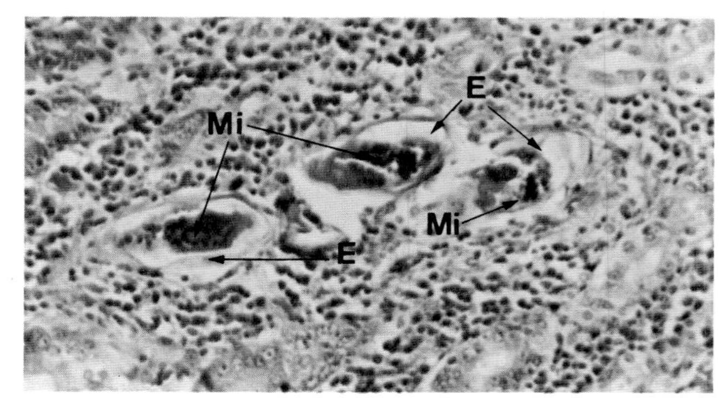

Gallbladder

This organ is seldom invaded by parasites. When it does occur it is usually an accidental infection, e.g., occupation of the lumen by a wandering *Clonorchis sinensis,* or penetration of the wall of the gallbladder by aberrant eggs of schistosomes.

Rotifera sp.

These minute organisms are not considered to be parasites of any animals. Massive experimental intravenous inoculation in laboratory animals revealed no evidence of pathogenicity. These organisms are included because one species has been found time and again in sections of various organs such as the stomach, lungs, brain, etc. Since these organisms usually breed in stagnant water it is possible that they are only pollutants of tissue sections introduced during laboratory processing.

Fig. 64. Ovum of *Schistosoma mansoni.*

A cross-sectioned egg (E) of *S. mansoni,* in the submucosal layer of the gallbladder, is completely calcified. There is a mild chronic inflammatory reaction around the calcified egg. The definite diagnosis of the species could not have been made without corroborative medical history and other laboratory examinations. (x400)

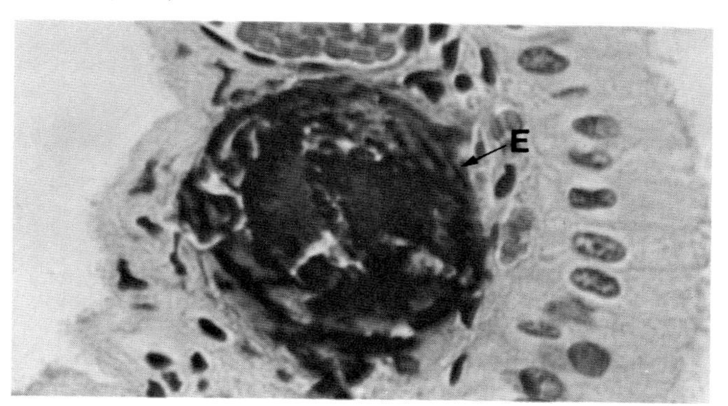

Fig. 63. Ova of *Schistosoma mansoni* in the gallbladder.

Remnants of two deformed eggshells (ES) of schistosomes in the submucosal fibromuscular layer of the gallbladder from a confirmed infection with *S. mansoni.* The mucosal epithelium is stripped away from the folds of the gallbladder. There is some congestion and lymphocytic infiltration. (x100)

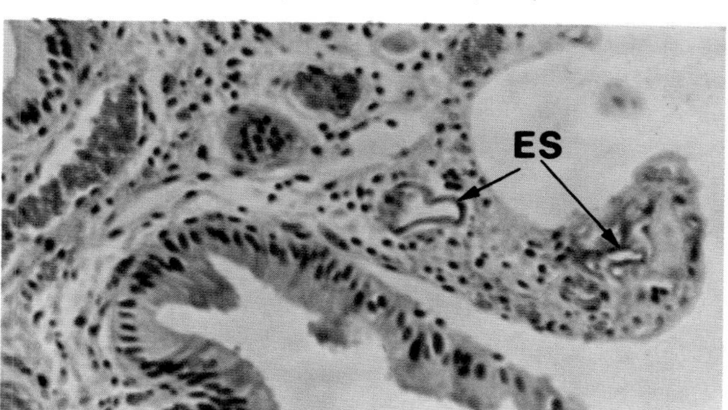

Fig. 65. Rotifera sp. in a section of the gallbladder.

The anterior spine of a *Rotifera* is stuck in the serous peritoneal layer of the gallbladder. The darkly stained organism (O) is within its chitinous lorica (L), an outer protective shell with a long anterior spine (AS) and a posterior crown of spines (PS). The fenestrated lorica allows one to see the organism filling its cavity. (x100)

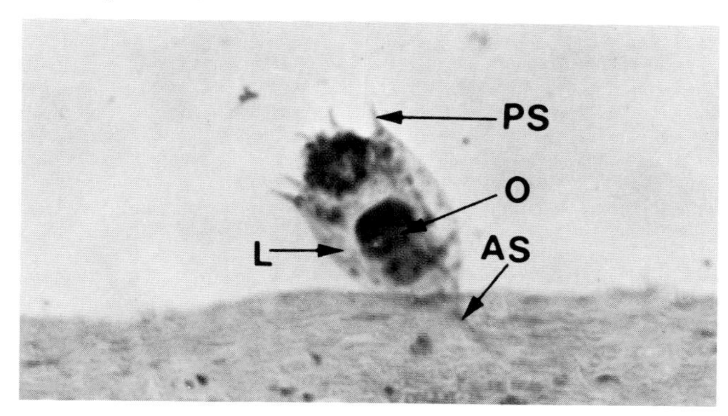

Urinary Bladder

The urinary bladder which is often involved in bacterial infections is usually affected by a single parasite, *Schistosoma haematobium.* However, the urinary bladder may be indirectly implicated in other parasitic infections, e.g., *Dioctophyme renale,* the kidney worm which in destroying the kidney may lead to infection of the urethra and the bladder. The female *Enterobius vermicularis* during its migration to the perianal region for the purpose of oviposition may accidentally make its way into the urinary bladder through the urethra. However, vesical schistosomiasis in which the urinary bladder has a part in the normal life cycle of *Schistosoma haematobium,* is the only parasitic infection routinely observed in tissue sections of that organ.

Schistosoma haematobium

As with the other blood flukes the distribution of this species of schistosomes is related to the presence of suitable snails as the intermediate hosts. The most important endemic area of bilharziasis is the Middle East but other significant foci of infection are in Africa and India. Man is the only important host and in some hyperendemic areas in Egypt up to 95 percent of the human population is infected. The eggs of *S. haematobium* as with the other two species of human schistosomes are the primary cause of pathogenesis. When passing from the perivesical venous plexus into the bladder the eggs engender damage that may range from an early inflammatory reaction and hematuria to progressive thickening, hyperplasia, and final fibrosis and ulcerations. As a result of constant irritation, carcinoma of the urinary bladder is not an infrequent complication. Ectopic eggs in distant organs are not as frequent in *S. haematobium* infection as they are in the other two species of schistosomes. However, the eggs of *S. haematobium* are commonly found in pelvic organs located in the proximity of the urinary bladder.

The eggs of *S. haematobium* measure 112-170/40-60 microns. They have a short, pointed terminal spine which because of its anatomical location can be seen only in longitudinal sections. When viable the eggs contain a miracidium.

Fig. 66. Eggs of *Schistosoma haematobium.*

Numerous eggs (E) of *S. haematobium* in the submucosa of the urinary bladder. Most are sectioned crosswise but occasionally eggs are seen in longitudinal section. The location of the eggs and their elongated form without the presence of a long lateral spine are sufficient for the diagnosis of this species. One egg, sectioned obliquely shows the typical short, terminal spine (S) characteristic of *S. haematobium.* (x100)

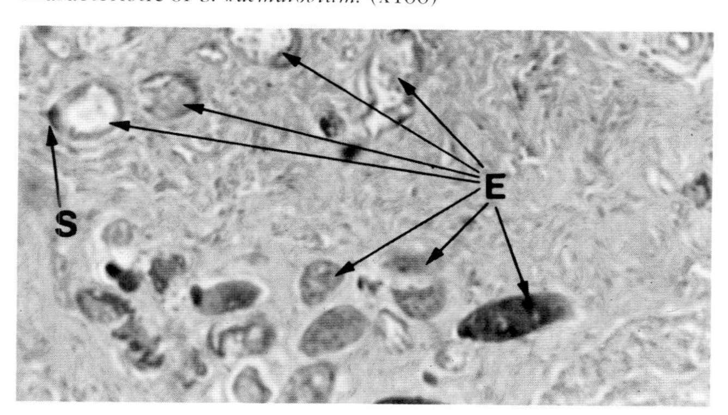

Fig. 67. Ova of *Schistosoma haematobium* in a biopsy of the urinary bladder.

In a vesical biopsy, there is a heavy infiltration of the submucosa by eggs (E) of *S. haematobium.* Practically all of the eggs are in longitudinal position. Some of them reveal the typical short, pointed, terminal spine (S). All the eggs have miracidia (Mi). (x100)

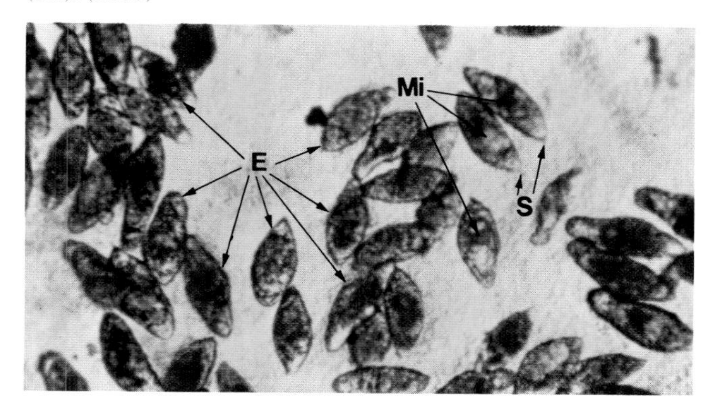

Fig. 68. Ova of *Schistosoma haematobium* in the urinary bladder with carcinoma.

Broken eggs (E) of *S. haematobium* are in the submucosa of the urinary bladder surrounded by a malignant proliferation (MP) of the bladder epithelium. One part of the egg, top, demonstrates the diagnostic short, terminal spine (TS) of this species. Each egg contains a miracidium (Mi). (x100)

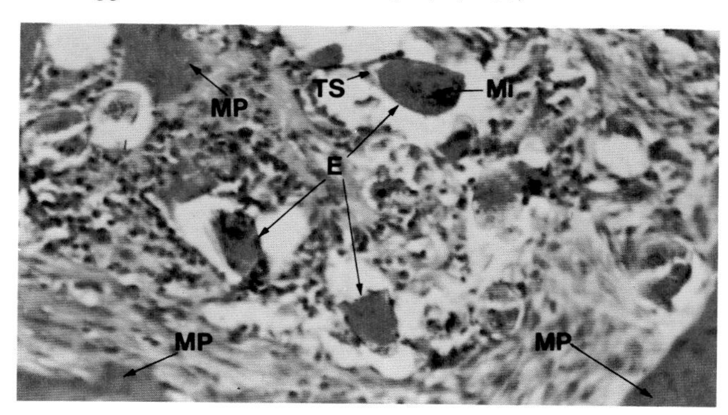

Fig. 69. Schistosoma haematobium in a perivesical vein.

Cross-section of an adult male (♂) of *S. haematobium* in a venule of the perivesical plexus. The parasite has only a slightly tuberculated integument (Int) as compared with the grossly tuberculated cuticle of *S. mansoni* and the absolutely smooth integument in *S. japonicum.* (x35)

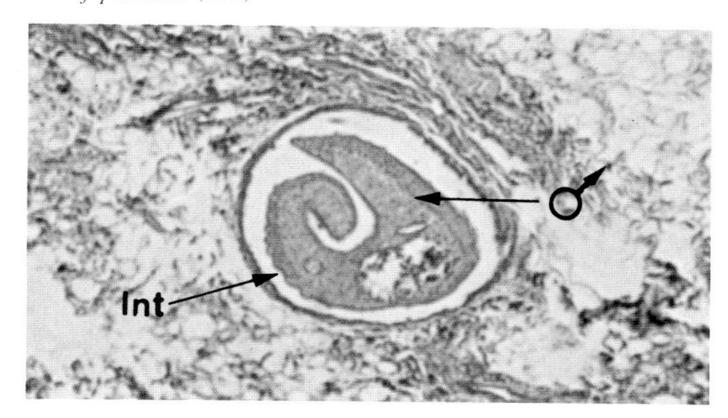

Lungs

The parasites found in tissue sections of the lungs are either accidental parasites, e.g., aberrant eggs of schistosomes or immature stages of parasites completing their life cycles within the human body, e.g., larvae of *Ascaris*. However, certain species such as *Paragonimus westermani* are true parasites of the lungs. Lung sections may occasionally reveal the presence of ectopic parasites which usually are harbored in other organs, e.g., amebae.

When a nematode larva is found in a tissue section of the lung, the differential diagnosis has to be made only between the larvae of *Ascaris*, hookworm and *Strongyloides*, the three nematode larvae migrating through the lung. The *Ascaris* larvae which undergo two molts in the lung and grow to 1,500 microns in length, are about twice as large as those of hookworm and *Strongyloides*.

Amebiasis of the lung

E. histolytica may invade the lung by direct extension from a hepatic abscess and in such a case it is usually found in the right lower lobe. It may also be found in any part of the lungs as a result of emboli originating from an amebic focus.

Fig. 70. Ovum of *Schistosoma mansoni* in the lung.

An egg (E) of *S. mansoni* sectioned in length in a granuloma (GR) of the lung shows its lateral spine (S) and a well perserved miracidium (Mi). (x100)

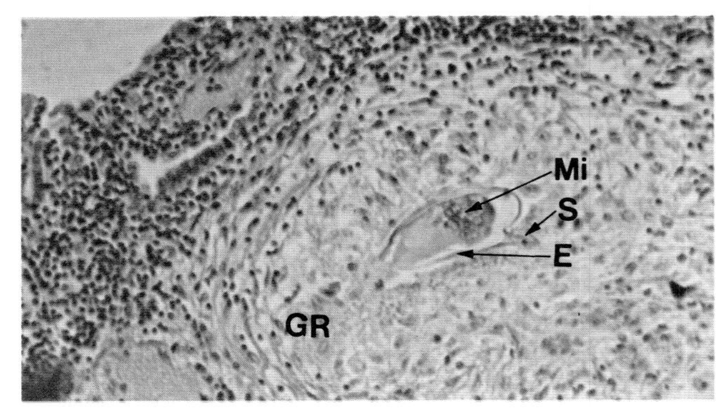

Fig. 71. Larvae of *Ascaris* in the lung.

Two larvae (L) of *Ascaris* in longitudinal sections in small bronchioles of the lung. There is edema and some consolidation of the lung. (x100)

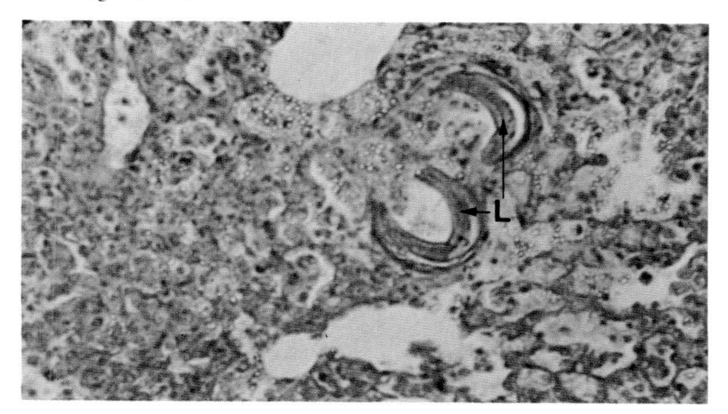

Fig. 72. Larvae of *Ascaris.*

Three larvae (L) of *Ascaris* are cross-sectioned in an alveolus of the lung. This higher magnification allows recognition of their typical long, muscle fibers (MF) under the cuticle (C) and the central digestive tract (DT). (x400)

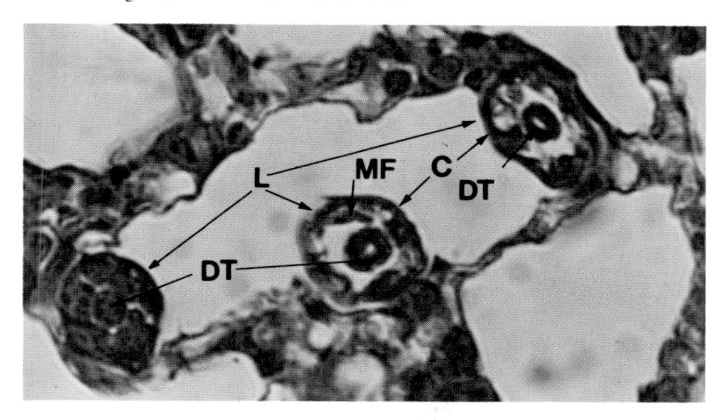

Fig. 73. Larvae of *Strongyloides stercoralis.*

One of numerous small granulomas (GR) of a lung in auto-infection with *S. stercoralis,* reveals small, round calcified bodies (CB) which represent the larvae in cross-section. (x40)

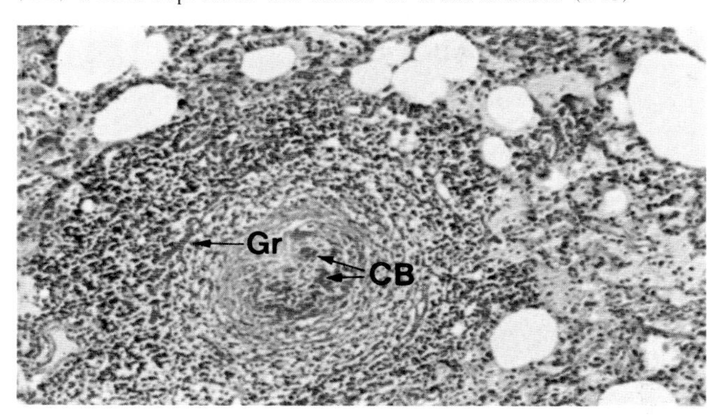

Fig. 74. Larva of *Strongyloides stercoralis.*

Part of a *S. stercoralis* larva (L), longitudinal section, during its passage through the lung, caused by auto-infection in strongyloidiasis. (x400)

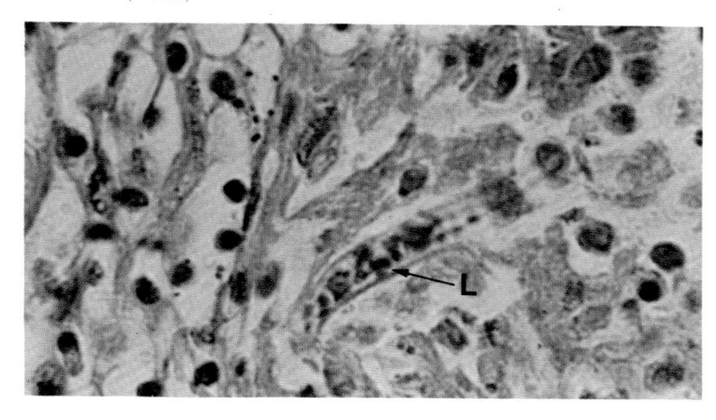

Fig. 75. Amebic abscess of the lung.

Three *E. histolytica* (E.h.) in a lung abscess. The amebae have the characteristic mottled appearance but not the diagnostic nucleus. There is some histolysis (H) of the lung around each ameba. (x400)

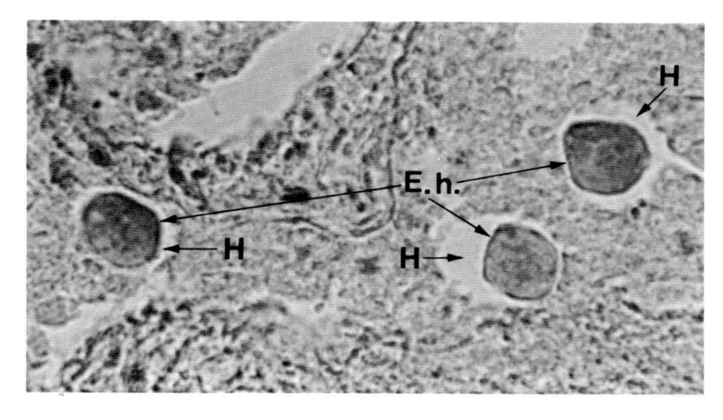

Fig. 76. *Entamoeba histolytica.*

Two *E. histolytica* (E.h.) surrounded by leukocytes in a section of sputum block, from a patient with a clinical diagnosis of carcinoma of the lung. One ameba shows the typical, large diagnostic nucleus (N) with its small central karyosome (K) and peripheral chromatin (PC). I. H. & E. (x1,000)

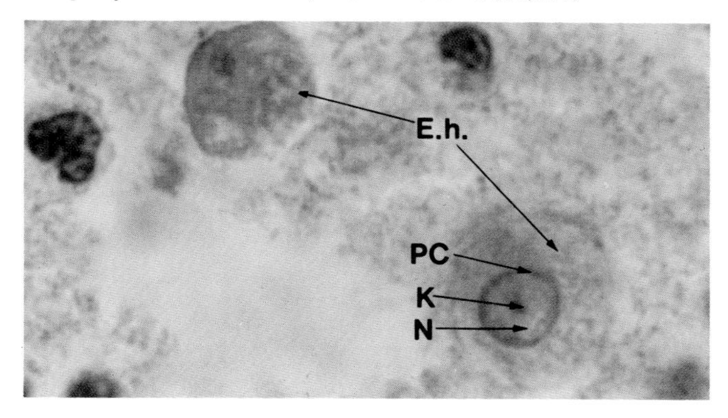

Paragonimus westermani (pulmonary fluke)

This is a large flat fluke measuring 8-16/4-8mm. It has a cosmopolitan distribution but is rarely found in North America. It has two intermediate hosts, one a suitable snail, the second either a crab or a crayfish. The infection is contracted by eating a second intermediate host harboring encysted metacercariae originating from the first intermediate host. The usual location of *P. westermani* is in the lung but aberrant parasites have been found in other locations. In the lung, the tissue reaction isolates the fluke within a thick, fibrous capsule containing hemorrhagic, perulent exudate and the eggs of the parasite. The golden-brown eggs measure 85/55 microns. They are very characteristic because of their thick rim into which the operculum fits.

Fig. 77. *Paragonimus* in the lung.

An adult *Paragonimus* (P) in cross-section within a thick fibrous capsule in the lung. The ventral sucker (VS) is on top, the large uterine cavity (UC) with occasional eggs (E) is to the right, and below it the ovary (O) and the flattened bladder (B). The small dark vitellaria (V) are in the lateral fields of the parasite. The lung (L) around the fibrous capsule (FC) is compressed. (x12)

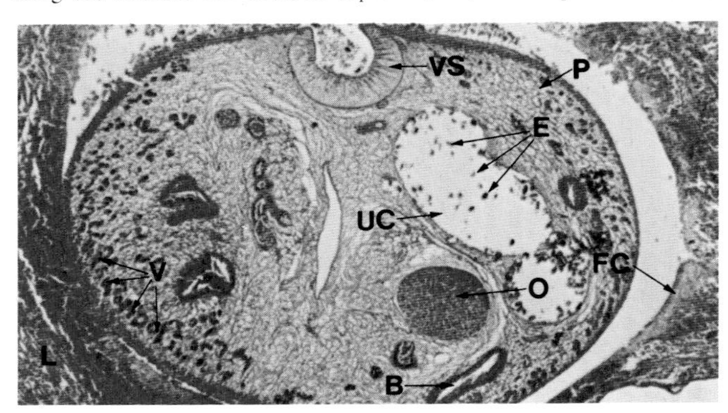

Fig. 78. Hydatid cyst of *Echinococcus granulosus.*

Part of the hydatid cyst in the lung demonstrates its typical structure. From left to right: the compressed, hemorrhagic lung (HL); the laminated cyst capsule (CAP) and, to the right of it, the darkly stained germinal layer (GL); on the extreme right, some coagulated hydatid fluid (Fl) within the cystic cavity. No scolices or hooklets are visible in this section. (x40)

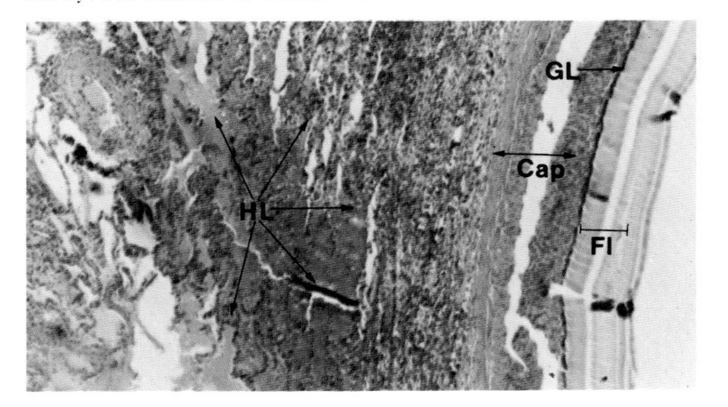

Pneumocystis carinii

P. carinii is a parasite of man as well as domestic and wild animals. These minute protozoa, measuring 1-2 microns, are extracellular parasites of the lungs and may be either free or within small cysts (7-9 microns). They are seldom recognized unless within a cyst which may contain up to eight parasites. Both the parasites and their cysts are strongly argyrophilic and any silver stain aids in their recognition. Pathologic changes of the lungs of the carriers may be minimal but they are marked in acute interstitial plasma cell pneumonia. The alveolar septa are usually thickened and infiltrated with a variety of inflammatory cells particularly plasma cells. The alveoli are filled with edema fluid and may become fibrosed.

Eosinophilic lung

An eosinophilic granuloma in the lung may be due to various causes. It may be the reaction to invasion by a visceral larva migrans or may represent an allergic response to *Strongyloides* larvae in auto-infection. It has also been described in tropical eosinophilia (Mayers and Kouwenaar syndrome, occult filariasis), in which microfilariae of *W. bancrofti* or *B. malayi* do not circulate in the blood but are destroyed in the organs. Sometimes an eosinophilic granuloma may be due to an accidental parasite such as *Linguatula serrata.* The adult of this arthropode is the parasite of the nasal cavities of carnivora in Europe, Africa and South America. Its four-legged larval stage is found in various organs of herbivorous animals but a number of infections with this stage have been reported in man. An eosinophilic granuloma may not reveal any parasite and systematic searching of numerous sections in the same area may be necessary.

Fig. 79. Brood capsule of *Echinococcus granulosus* in hydatid sand.

A brood capsule (BC) in a hydatid cyst detached from the germinal layer, contains invaginated scolices (S). (x100)

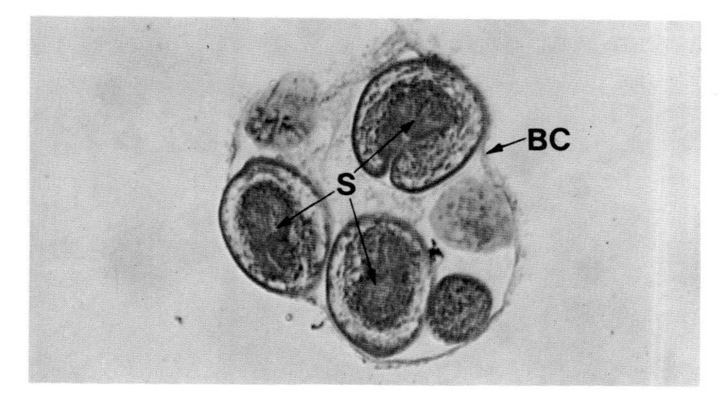

Fig. 80. *Pneumocystis carinii* in the lung.

One diagnostic cyst of *P. carinii* (P.c.) containing eight parasites stained blue, center, in an imprint made with lung tissue. Giemsa. (x900)

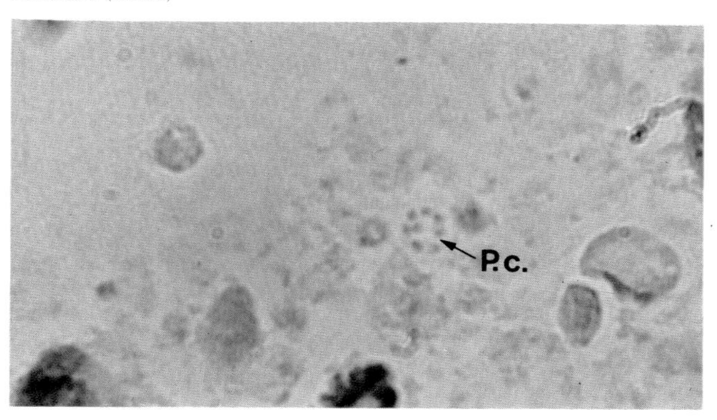

Fig. 81. *Pneumocystis carinii* in the lung.

Numerous cysts (C) of *P. carinii* in early stages within the edema fluid (EF) in an alveolus of the lung. Some cysts appear empty, others contain one or two protozoa (P) stained blue-black. Gomeri methenamine silver. (x1,000)

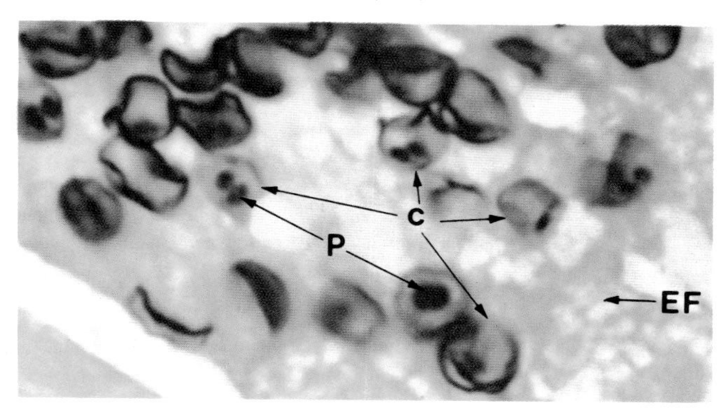

Fig. 82. Eosinophilic granuloma.

A typical eosinophilic granuloma (EG) in the lung, in a case of tropical eosinophilia. (x400)

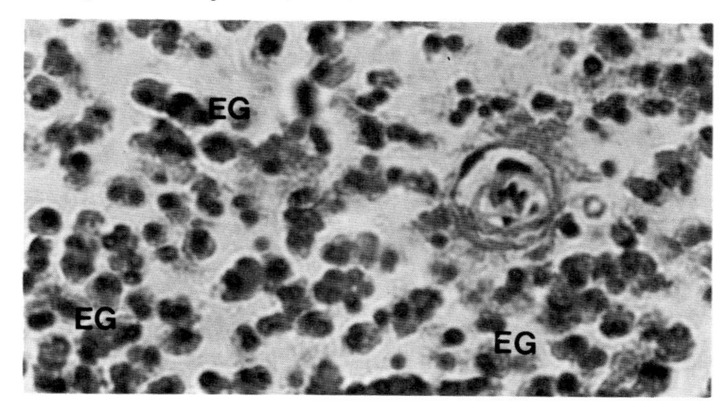

Fig. 83. *Linguatula serrata* in the lung.

The four-legged acariform embryo (E) of *L. serrata* is in a granuloma containing numerous eosinophiles in the lung. Part of one leg (L) can be seen on top and to the right of the parasite. (x400)

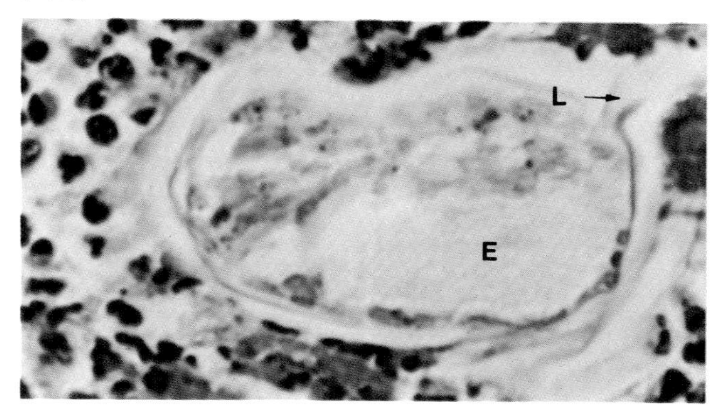

Heart

Fig. 84. Malarial pigment in the heart.
The dark deposits of hemozoin (H), the malarial pigment, are partially blocking the capillaries of the heart in a case of *P. falciparum* infection. (x100)

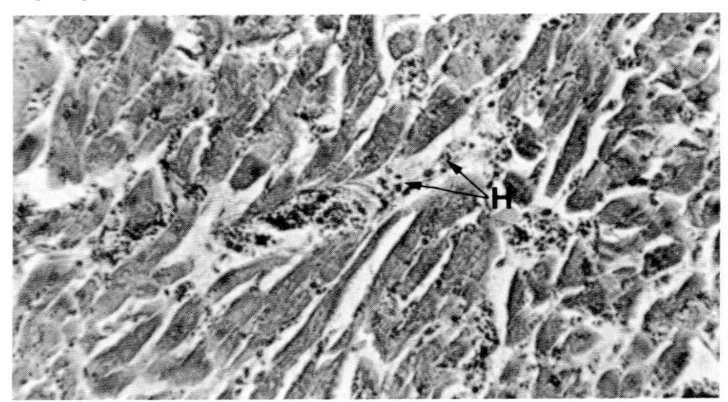

Fig. 85. Leishmanial stage of *Trypanosoma cruzi.*
The mass of leishmanian forms of *T. cruzi* in the myocardial cell is very compact, perhaps more so than usually found in a cell invaded by *Leishmania.* There are numerous rod-shaped kinetoplasts (K) clearly visible near the larger, rounded nuclei (N) of the parasites. The heart muscle shows evidence of severe myocarditis even in this early stage of Chagas' disease. (x900)

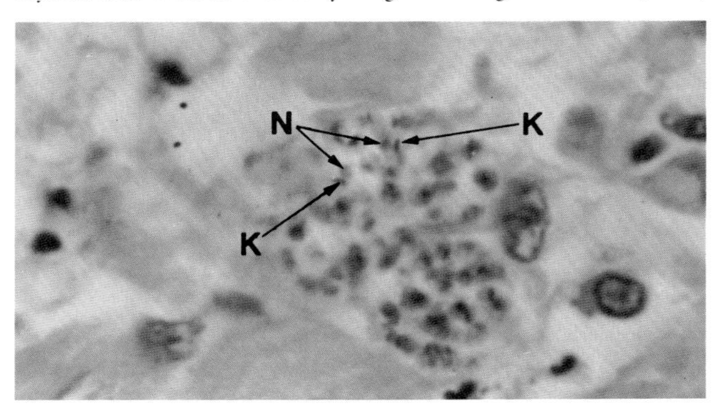

Larvae of many species of parasites pass through the heart during their normal life cycles, e.g., larvae of *Ascaris, Strongyloides,* hookworm, etc. Usually such larvae do not invade the myocardium. Larvae of *Trichinella spiralis* which have a special predilection for striated muscles may penetrate the myocardium but they soon disintegrate and are absorbed. For all practical purposes, only three species of parasites should be sought in examining heart sections: the plasmodia of malaria, the leishmanian forms of Chagas' disease and the *Toxoplasma* organisms.

Malaria

The heart is affected most in *P. falciparum* infections. In heavy infections, sections of the heart reveal a marked congestion of the capillaries often blocked by infected erythrocytes and malarial pigment. There may be evidence of anoxemia, with changes varying from cloudy swelling and fatty degeneration to myocardial infarctions. With the other three species of malaria, heart sections are not remarkable except for congestion of the capillaries.

Chagas' disease (American trypanosomiasis)

This disease is found in South and Central America and occasionally in Southern Mexico. Man and other vertebrate animals are the hosts of the parasite, *Trypanosoma cruzi* and transmission is made by reduviid bugs. The parasite of *Chagas' disease* assumes two forms within the host. *T. cruzi,* a typical trypanosome, can be found in the peripheral blood, while in organs the parasite assumes a leishmanian form similar to that of *L. donovani.* Although the leishmanian form of *T. cruzi* may invade any organ, preferably reticuloendothelial macrophages, many strains have a special predilection for the cardiac muscles. The invasion of the heart may lead to severe myocardial damage and death.

Fig. 86. Toxoplasmosis. *Toxoplasma gondii* in the heart.
A cyst (C) of *T. gondii* in a longitudinal section of a heart muscle fiber, shows its tightly packed organisms, their nuclei (N) of even size, and the absence of kinetoplasts. (x1,000)

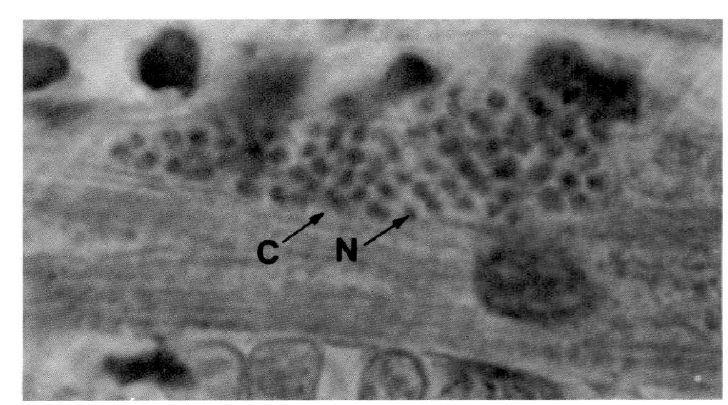

Skeletal Muscles

Among the parasites which invade the voluntary muscles, only four species are of importance: *Trichinella spiralis, Sarcocystis lindemani, Toxoplasma gondii* and *Cysticercus cellulosae.*

Trichinella spiralis

This disease is by far the most important and frequent parasitic infection of the striated muscles. Trichinosis has a world-wide distribution and any carnivorous animal may be infected. Although the host harbors both the adult and larval stages, two hosts are required to accomplish the life cycle. The intermediate host in human infection is the pig and therefore, the incidence among the orthodox Jews

Fig. 87. Trichinella spiralis larvae.
The pressed, unstained muscle removed by biopsy shows a small coiled larva (L) of *T. spiralis.* There is already evidence of a capsule (Cap) formation around the larva. Unstained. (x25)

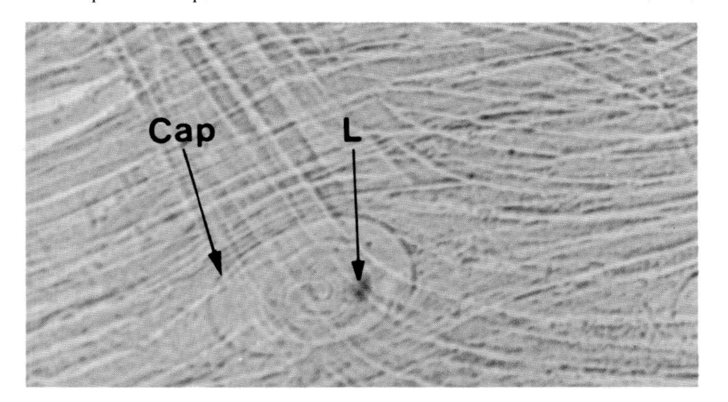

Fig. 89. Trichinella spiralis larvae.
The larvae (L) of *T. spiralis* encysted in muscle fibers (MF) are older than the larva in Figure 88. The larva seen in longitudinal section preserves its transverse striation but the capsules (Cap) are thicker. The inflammatory reaction is minimal. (x100)

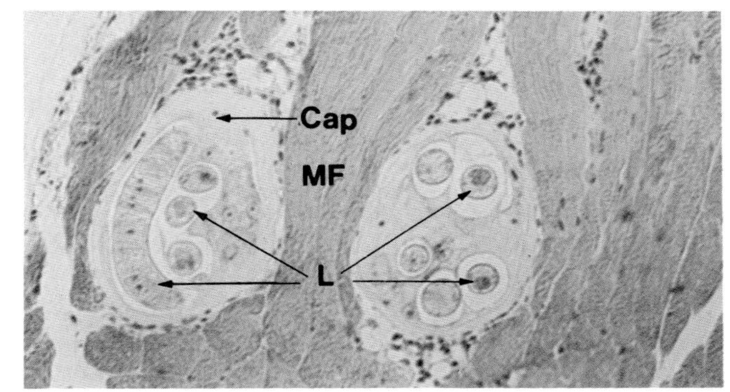

Fig. 88. Trichinella spiralis larva in muscle.
The larva (L) of *T. spiralis* appears in both longitudinal and cross-section. Edema (E) and cellular infiltration (CI) mark the borders of the capsule starting to form around the larva. (x100)

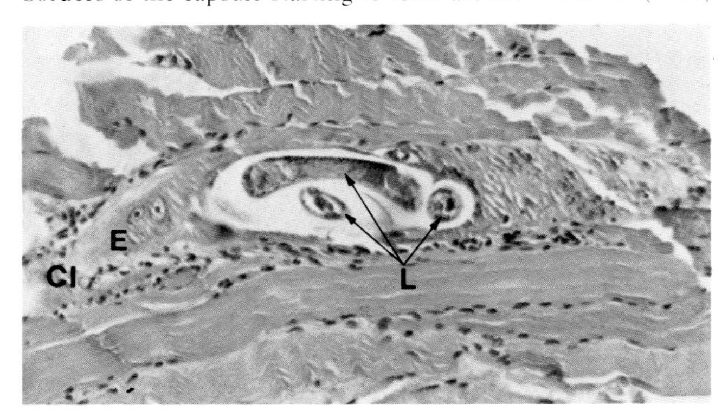

Fig. 90. Trichinella spiralis larva in muscle.
The larva (L) of *T. spiralis* is well preserved, as evidenced by its morphological structure, visible in cross-sections. The muscle fiber (MF) is characteristically distended and has lost its striated appearance in the process of degeneration. (x100)

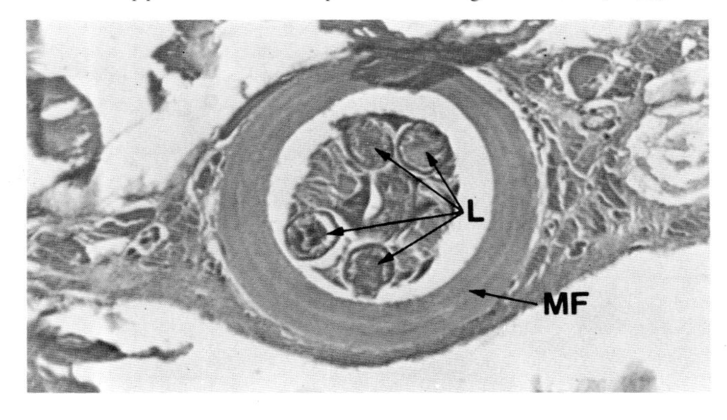

and the Mohammedans is very low. Neither is the infection rate high among people who eat only well cooked pork, e.g., the Puerto Ricans.

After raw trichinous pork is consumed, the larvae emerge from the cysts and develop in the small intestine of the new host into adult males and females measuring 1.5-3.5/0.04-0.06mm., the female being the larger. The adult *T. spiralis* is practically never found in tissue sections. Forty-eight hours after the infection, the female starts to deposit larvae deep within the mucosa of the small intestine. A single female may release up to 1,500 larvae in six weeks. These larvae may reach any organ through the systemic circulation but are able to encyst and survive only in the striated skeletal muscles. Therefore, *T. spiralis* is found only in such tissue sections. The diaphragm is most frequently invaded. On post-mortem over 15 percent of the diaphragms examined in the United States have been estimated to be infected. Biopsies are usually made in the most accessible places on muscles near tendinous attachments such as the gastrocnemius, deltoid or the biceps. Because the larvae do not coil until the seventeenth day of the infection the biopsy is usually not made before the third week.

The larva of *T. spiralis* resembles the adults. It is tapering toward the anterior end, has a crosswise striation, measures only 5.6 microns when deposited, but grows rapidly within the muscle to sometimes attain over 1,000/35 microns. The invaded muscle fiber undergoes inflammation and degeneration. The capsule formed around the parasite is the result of tissue reaction. During the growth of the larva the muscle fiber undergoes considerable distension which persists even after the larva dies and is calcified.

Sarcocystis lindemani

There is no general agreement on the classification, nature and the life cycle of this parasite. Numerous species are found in mammals, birds and reptiles. Man may be only an accidental host and the human species, *S. lindemani*, morphologically is similar to the animal parasites. The infection is probably acquired by injestion of sporocysts eliminated in the feces of infected animals. The parasite establishes itself in striated muscles forming cylindrical cysts called Miescher's tubes. They have a double outer membrane and transverse trabeculae separating the cystic cavity into closed compartments. These small chambers are packed with spores of *Sarcocystis* varying in size, 10-16/4-7 microns with the largest spores located in the center of the cyst. The Miescher's

Fig. 91. Calcified larva of *Trichinella spiralis.*
A very old, calcified larva (L) of *T. spiralis* is not easy to recognize in a degenerated muscle fiber. It is possible to make out the rounded contours of the. cross-sectioned larva within the calcified area and the characteristically distended muscle fiber (MF). (x100)

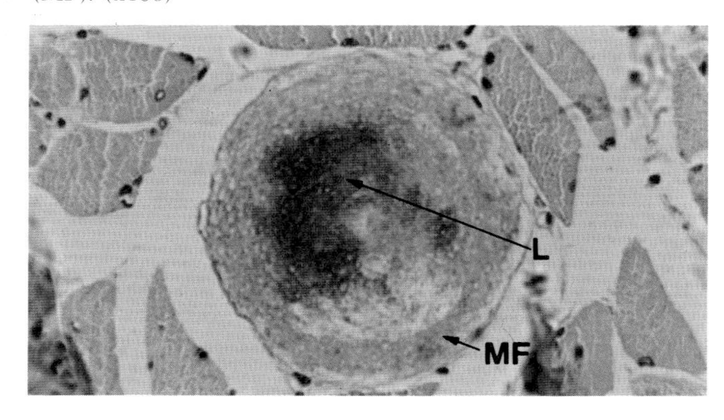

Fig. 92. Sarcocystis in muscle.
Two Miescher's tubes (MT) in muscle fibers (MF) are sectioned longitudinally. Neither fills the whole cell but leaves the borders of the muscle free, just as the *Toxoplasma* cyst does. The outside thin capsule and the internal dividing septa cannot be seen in this section. The darkly stained crescentic spores fill the cysts. (x100)

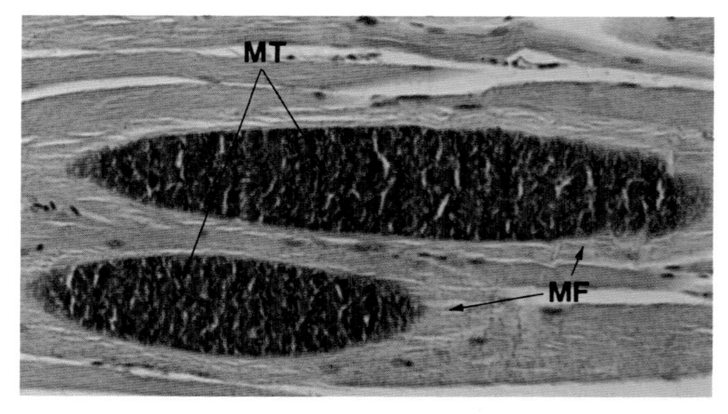

tube in cross-section somewhat resembles the cyst of toxoplasma. However, the organisms of *Sarcocystis* are more sickle-shaped and larger. The external capsule and the internal dividing septa of *Sarcocystis*, not present in *T. gondii*, are not always visible when the section is routinely stained with hematoxylin and eosin but are very argyrophilic, i.e., clearly visible with any silver staining method.

Except for the damage to the invaded muscle fiber, pathogenesis is only important in very heavy infections and is due to the toxins derived from *Sarcocystis*.

Cysticercus cellulosae

The larval stage of *Taenia solium*, the *C. cellulosae*, is usually found in the pig, the intermediate host of this large tapeworm. Cysticercosis is acquired by swallowing an egg of *T. solium* in contaminated food or water. Man can also get infected with *Cysticercus* larvae by autoinfection while harboring the adult worm of *T. solium*. This may occur either by accidental ingestion of the *Taenia* eggs due to poor individual hygiene or when the eggs in the small intestine are carried to the stomach by regurgitation and reversed peristalsis. Whichever way the eggs of *T. solium* reach the stomach of man, their outer shells are dissolved. The *Cysticercus* larvae at this stage called onchospheres, hatch from the eggs in the small intestine, penetrate its wall, and are carried by the bloodstream to practically any organ in the body. The occurrence of *C. cellulosae* in the various organs as established by post mortem examination is as follows: brain, eye, muscles, heart, liver, lungs and even the abdominal cavity, where *Cysticercus* larvae may be found in tissue sections.

C. cellulosae is an oval or rounded cyst containing an invaginated scolex with its crown of hooklets and four suckers. At maturity which is attained within 2 to 3 months, the cyst measures about 5 mm. in diameter but in the soft brain tissue may grow larger. Except for the brain and the vitreous of the eye, the *Cysticercus* larva is usually surrounded by a capsule resulting from tissue reaction. The cystic membrane is usually wrinkled after laboratory processing giving the cyst a folded appearance. This folding is so characteristic as to be diagnostic even when the scolex is not present in the section.

The gravity of the infection depends upon the location of *C. cellulosae* and is related to the number of cysts. When cysticercosis is due to repeated infections, or to regurgitation of a gravid proglottid of *T. solium* containing thousands of eggs, the cysts may be extremely numerous.

Fig. 93. *Sarcocystis* in muscle.

Part of a cyst of *Sarcocystis* demonstrates its peripheral capsule (Cap) and multiple internal septa (Sep) dividing the cyst into compartments. (x100)

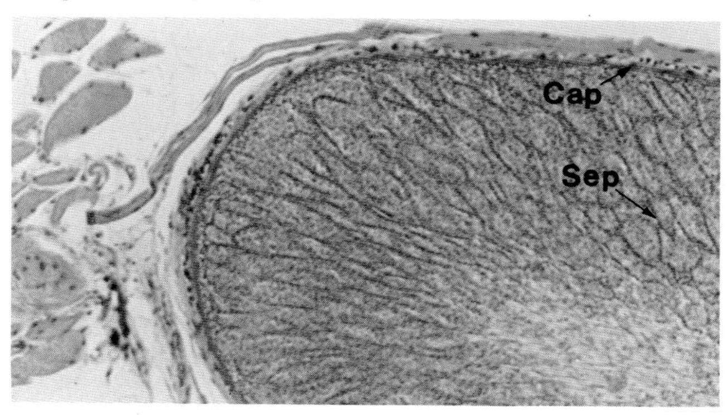

Fig. 94. *Sarcocystis* in muscle.

The thin outer capsule of *Sarcocystis* is visible on the cyst under high magnification. Most of the spores (Sp), left, are sectioned longitudinally and many demonstrate their crescentic shape. In the right lower corner, there are polymorphonuclear leukocytes (Leuk) near a muscle fiber (MF). (x540)

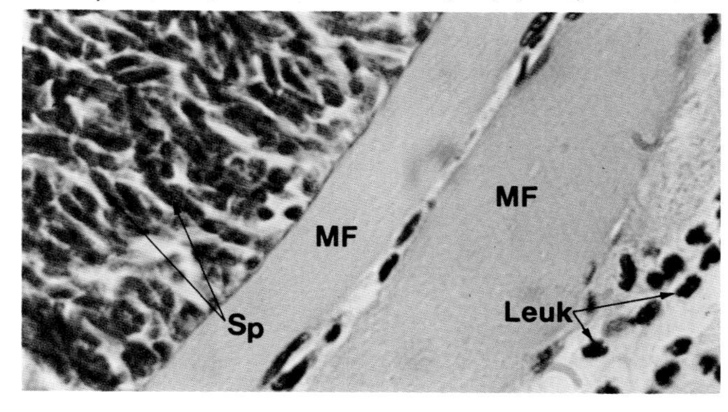

Fig. 95. *Cysticercus cellulosae* in muscle.

The typical folding of the capsule (Cap) covering the bladder and the mazelike network of folds are characteristic in this *C. cellulosae* located within the muscle (M). Part of the scolex (S) is visible with two of its four suckers, but no hooklets are present. To the left, adipose (A) tissue. (x12)

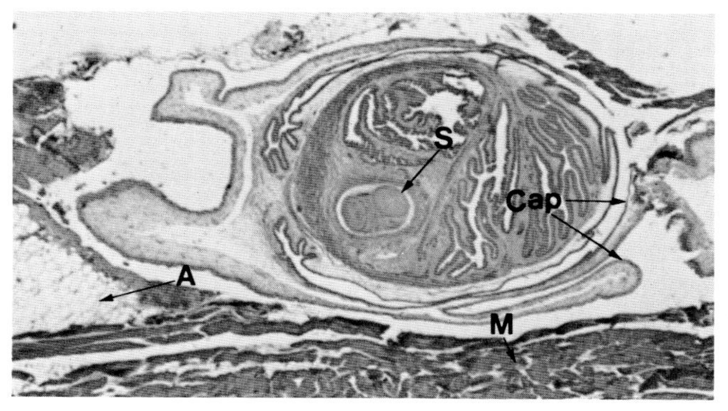

Skin and Subcutaneous Tissue

The human skin is invaded by various types of parasites. It may serve as a port of entry for parasites which can then enter the blood vessels and be carried to their permanent location, e.g., schistosomes, hookworms. Other parasites have a predilection for the skin itself. Among those are some insects or mites which use the skin for their ovipositon, e.g., the sand flea. Others are protozoa, like those of *Leishmania* sp., or nematodes which include the filaria worms producing onchocerciasis. Some parasites which may establish themselves in other locations also invade the subcutaneous tissue, e.g., sparganum larva. Because of this range of parasitic infestation the damage to the skin may vary from minimal and temporary to severe and permanent.

Sparganosis

Man may be infected by a larval stage of Spirometra, a tapeworm of lower animals. This infection occurs primarily in the Far East but is found to a lesser degree all over the world, even including the Americas. The adult *Spirometra* resembles *Diphyllobothrium latum*, the fish tapeworm of man, except that it is smaller. The life cycle of both parasites follows the same pattern. *Spirometra* needs two intermediate hosts. The first is a *Cyclops*, a small crustacean, which carries the procercoid larva derived from an egg of the tapeworm. The second intermediate hosts are frogs, snakes and small mammals. These second intermediate hosts, by swallowing an infected *Cyclops*, develop the next larval stage of the tapeworm, the plerocercoid larva, also called sparganum larva. By swallowing this larva an animal completes the life cycle and develops an adult *Spirometra*. Man usually acquires spraganosis by swallowing an infected *Cyclops* and harboring the sparganum larva. Man can also be infected by consuming the raw or undercooked flesh of a secondary intermediate host, such as a frog, already infected with sparganosis. In some areas of the world the use of poultices containing the infected flesh of a frog allows the sparganum larvae to crawl into the cutaneous lesion and gain entrance into a human host. Once in man, the sparganum larvae often invade the subcutaneous tissue or the muscles. They may also be found in or about the eyes, although they may invade practically any viscera and can be found in tissue sections. The presence of sparganum larvae

Fig. 96. Sparganosis in the subcutaneous tissue.
Part of sparganum larva (L) is visible. The smooth, undulating cuticle (C), the thin layer of muscle fibers (MF) underneath it, stained red, and the loose stroma containing bluish calcareous corpuscles (BCC) of various sizes are typical of an adult tapeworm in which this sparganum larva would develop if it were harbored in a suitable host. (x40)

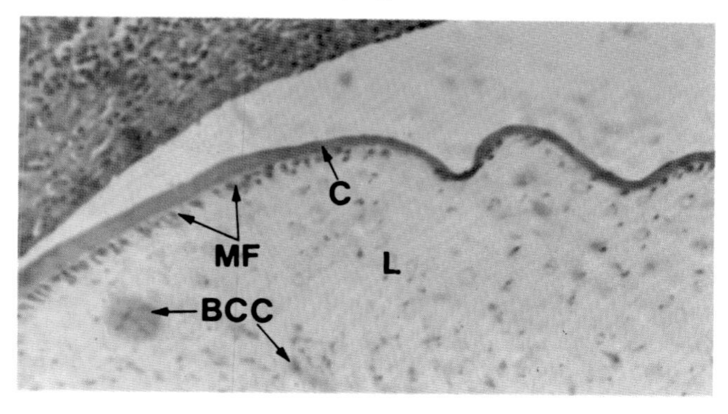

Fig. 97. Demodex folliculorum.
A sebaceous gland (SG) of the skin is invaded by three mites (M) of *D. folliculorum.* A long, worm-like abdomen (Ab) of one mite can be seen deep within the gland on the left side. The acanthotic epidermis (Ep) lines the gland deep into the dermis. There are some chronic inflammatory cells around the skin appendage. (x40)

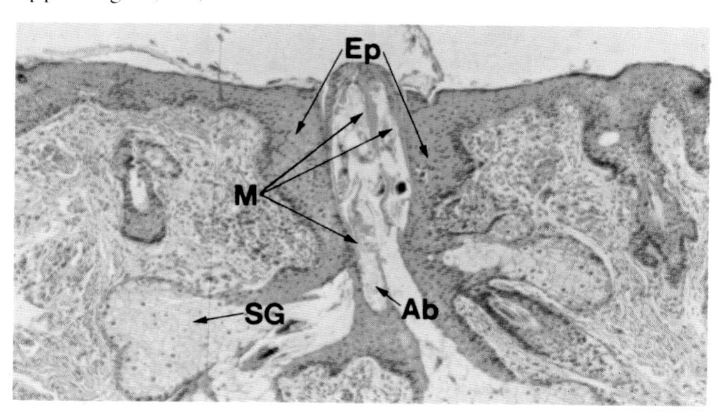

usually results in an acute inflammatory reaction which is even more intense after the larva dies and is absorbed. An even more severe reaction is produced by *Sparganum proliferum,* the larval stage of a pseudophyllidian tapeworm, the adult form being unknown. This larva characteristically branches off resulting in new sparganum larvae in the tissue.

Demodex folliculorum

This cosmopolitan parasite invades hair follicles and sebaceous glands of man and domestic animals. It has been found in the skin of every part of the human body including the eyelashes. Sometimes, two or three mites may infect the same sebaceous gland. The mite has four pairs of short legs attached to the anterior thoracic part and a long worm-like body. These mites seldom cause discomfort but conditions such as chronic erythema, acne, keratitis, etc., have been attributed to infestation by this parasite.

Scabies

This is a cosmopolitan infection of many mammals affecting the superficial layer of the skin. *Sarcoptes scabiei* is the parasite of man only. It is an oval, dorsally convex mite, measuring 200-450 microns, the female being almost twice the size of the male. The mites have four pairs of short legs and are ornamented with various chitinous processes. After copulation which takes place on the surface of the skin the female burrows deep into the corneous layer of the skin for oviposition in the tunnels it has excavated, but never below the epidermis. The preferential sites are the interdigital spaces but in heavy infestations the skin of the whole body can be involved, including the genitalia. The lesions

Fig. 98. Scabies in the skin.
This section contains two large females (♀) of *Sarcoptes scabiei* in deep tunnels within the stratum granulosum of the skin. Characteristically, these parasites do not invade the dermis (D). Chitinous remnants of a small male (♂) can be seen in the superficial layer of the epidermis. There are some chronic inflammatory cells within the dermis. (x100)

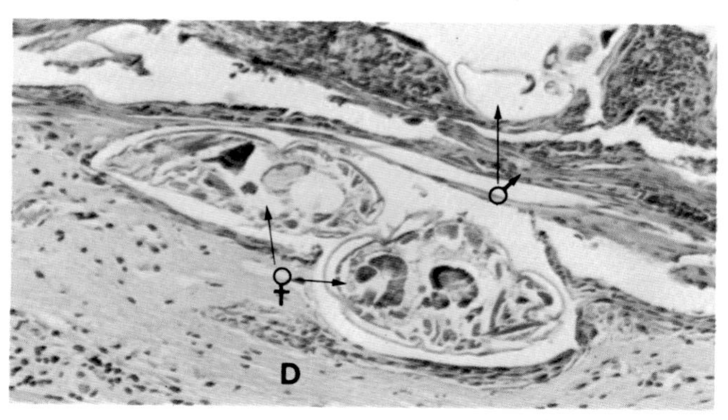

observed in tissue sections usually reveal not only those produced by the parasites but also the results of scratching induced by itching and often by a secondary bacterial infection. In some sections the parasite itself is not visible but only their burrows containing eggs and feces of the mites.

Tunga penetrans (Chigoe, sand flea)

This burrowing flea is the parasite of man and dog in tropical America and Africa. It is a very small flea not exceeding 1mm. After being impregnated the female flea burrows itself into the skin and becomes tremendously distended by its eggs. It has a predilection for the toes but may invade other locations, even the soles of the feet which are too tough to be penetrated by mites. The presence of *T. penetrans* produces an intense itching, even pain, and the flea is usually removed at this early stage. If it is left in the skin until the oviposition time the flea shrinks to its normal size and falls out through an exit left open, leaving the eggs behind. The attempts to remove a sand flea full of eggs may result in rupturing the flea, which often causes a secondary infection, occasionally leading to the loss of toes.

Filariasis

Man may harbor nine species of filarial worms: *Wuchereria bancrofti, Brugia malayi, Loa loa, Onchocerca volvulus, Acanthocheilonema perstans, Mansonella ozzardi, Dipetalonema streptocerca, Dirofilaria immitis* and *Dirofilaria tenuis.* The adult filaria measure 23-500/0.07-0.50mm. depending on their species and sex. Their location also varies with the species. The adults of *W. bancrofti* and *B. malayi* inhabit the lymphatic vessels; *Loa loa* migrates almost constantly in the subcutaneous tissues but the worms

Fig. 99. Tunga penetrans in the skin.

An impregnated female of *T. penetrans* in cross-section of a burrow made within the keratinized stratum granulosum of the skin. Some eggs (E) are within the cavity limited by the chitinous surface (CS) of the sand flea. (x12)

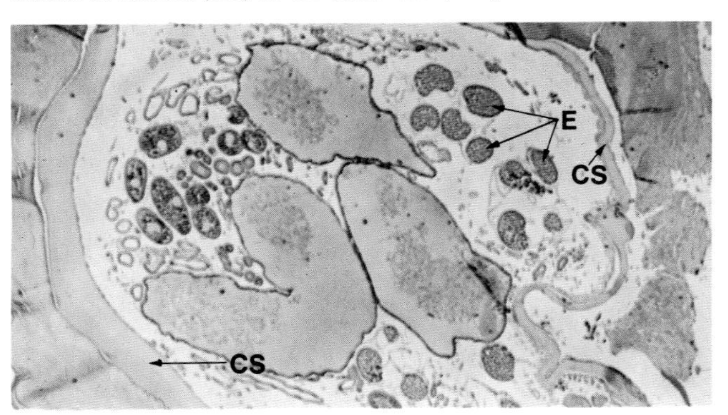

Fig. 100. Hookworm larvae in the skin.

The infective filariform hookworm larvae (HL) in both longitudinal and cross-sections within the skin. The only differential diagnosis of nematode larvae in this location should be made with larvae of *Strongyloides,* which is not possible in skin sections. (x100)

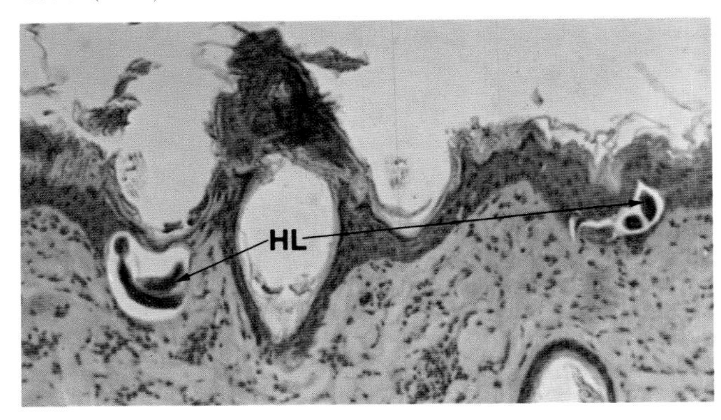

Fig. 101. Leishmania tropica
(oriental sore, cutaneous leishmaniasis).

No *Leishmania* organisms can be recognized at this low magnification. The epidermis (Epid) shows slight acanthosis, but no ulcerations. There is evidence of diffuse edema and round cell infiltration in the corium (C). Areas of collagen formation point to a focal regeneration. (x40)

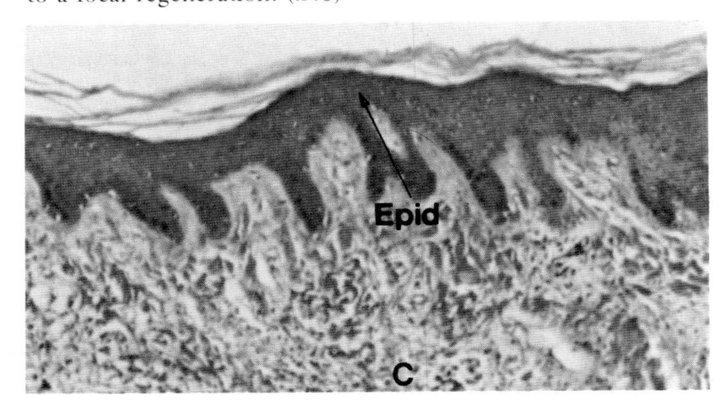

Fig. 102. Leishmania tropica.

Groups of *Leishmania tropica* (L.t.) organisms seen with oil immersion objective in the edematous dermis of the skin. Some of the *Leishmania* demonstrate an oval nucleus (N) and the diagnostic, linear kinetoplast (K). Occasionally, only the nucleus or the kinetoplast is visible. The dermis is infiltrated with phagocytes. Giemsa. (x1,000)

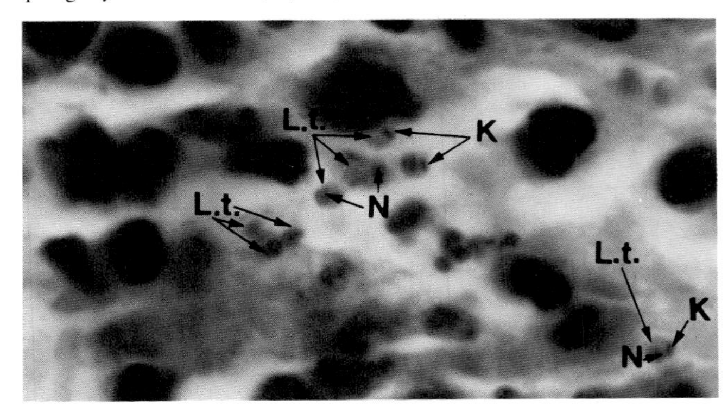

occasionally wander into various viscera; *O. volvulus* is found in subcutaneous nodules; and both *A. perstans* and *M. ozzardi* inhabit body cavities: the abdominal cavity, pleural cavity and the pericardium. For all practical purposes *D. perstans* and *M. ozzardi* are never found in tissue sections and the diagnosis must be made by finding microfilariae in the peripheral blood smears. In infections with *O. volvulus* and *D. streptocerca* microfilariae may be found not in blood smears but in skin sections.

Onchocerca volvulus

This filarial worm has no definitive host other than man. It has a vast range in Africa, Central America, and the northern part of South America. Its geographical distribution is related to the presence of the intermediate host, the *Simulium* sp., black fly. The male worm measures 19-42/0.13-0.21mm. while the females are much larger and attain up to 500/0.40mm. Both sexes invade and coil in subcutaneous tissues which soon become hard, fibrous nodules. These nodules of African onchocerciasis are located on the trunk or near bony prominences while most of the nodules seen in patients in Guatemala and Southern Mexico are on the head. The location of nodules has an important clinicopathological implication. Microfilariae of other species of filarial worms circulate freely in the blood while those of *O. volvulus* remain in the skin. When the nodules are located on the head, microfilariae of *O. volvulus* can invade the cornea and other functional parts of the eyes which may result in blindness. The fibrous nodules which may number from 1 to over 100 often become caseous and calcified. In sections, all adult filarial worms are very similar. However, certain criteria such as location in a skin nodule and not a lymph vessel, help the differential diagnosis between *O. volvulus* and *W. bancrofti.* Such a diagnosis is more difficult in old infections, when due to tissue shrinkage the worms in onchoceriasis appear to lie within small vessels, while no lymphatic fluid is recognizable in old *Wuchereria* infections. When there are many worms in cross-section, all in one cavity, it is probably *W. bancrofti* in a lymph vessel, even though the lining endothelium cannot be recognized. If there are many worms, each in a small cavity, this is an artifact produced by retraction of connective tissue around each *Onchocerca.* Another diagnostic aid in onchocerciasis is the presence of microfilariae in skin nodules and not in dermis as in streptocerciasis. The microfilariae of *O. volvulus* measure 150-368/5-9 microns. They have no external sheaths and the extremities are free from small nuclei that fill the rest of the microfilariae.

Fig. 103. Onchocerca volvulus.

The fibrous skin nodule (SN) contains multiple adult *O. volvulus.* Each cross-section of the filaria worm occupies a small space formed by retraction of connective tissue around the parasites. Examination under high magnification would confirm the absence of endothelium lining these spaces and the presence of microfilariae in the tissue around the adults. Typically, adult females appear with paired uteri (U) containing either rounded ova or worm-like microfilariae (M). (x35)

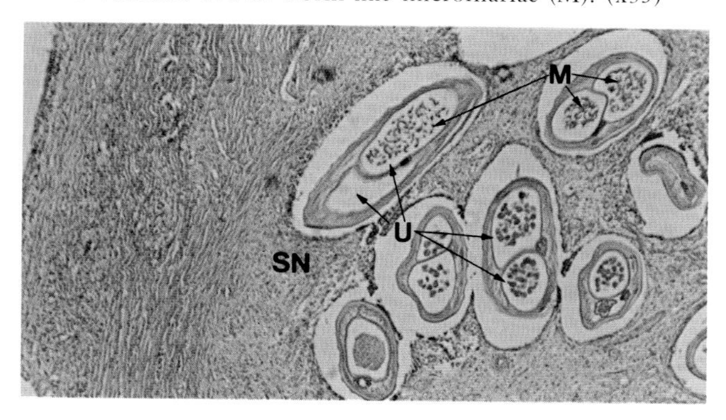

Fig. 104. Onchocerca volvulus in a skin nodule.

A cross-section of an adult female of *O. volvulus* (♀ O.v.) demonstrates its characteristic bilateral uteri (U) containing calcified eggs (CE) and the digestive tract (DT) below. An atrophied, hyalinized vein is below the parasite. (x100)

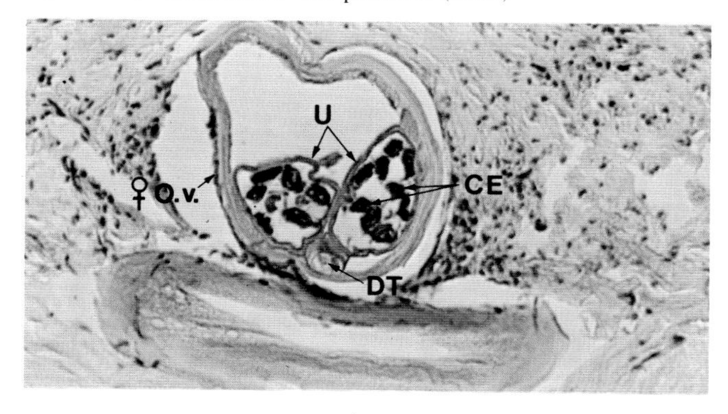

Fig. 105. Microfilaria of *Onchocerca volvulus* in a skin nodule.

A relatively new nodule contains a coiled microfilaria (M) of *O. volvulus.* (x400)

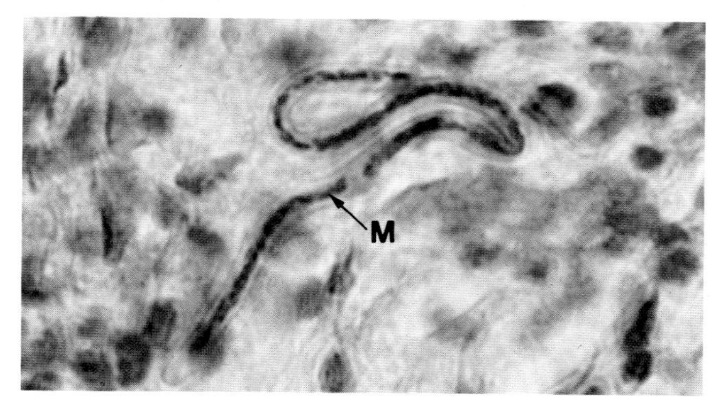

Lymphatic Vessels

Larval stages of many parasites use the lymphatic circulation as well as the bloodstream to reach their destination during their migration within the body of the host. However, they are rarely found in tissue sections. Those found are parasites that actually live within the lymphatic channels, e.g., *Wuchereria bancrofti.*

Wuchereria bancrofti

The parasite of bancroftian filariasis has a fairly world-wide distribution but is limited to tropical and subtropical areas. It measures 40-83/0.10-0.24 mm., the female being larger. These parasites live within the human host about five years but the damage such as elephantiasis may last long after the death of the worms. The parasites may not be found within the tissues for years after the initial infection even when allergic sensitization points to their presence in the lymphatic system. On the other hand, *W. bancrofti* may be found in the lymphatics years after the worms have died. The damage to the human host ranges from inflammatory sensitization to elephantiasis. Elephantiasis is due to both the allergic response of the host and the mechanical obstruction of the lymphatics.

Fig. 106. Wuchereria bancrofti in lymphatic vessels.
Numerous filarial worms of both sexes are visible in cross-section. The females of *W. bancrofti* (♀W.b.) demonstrate the characteristic picture of bilateral uteri (U). The lymph (Ly) within the vessel lined with endothelium confirms the diagnosis of the species. (x35)

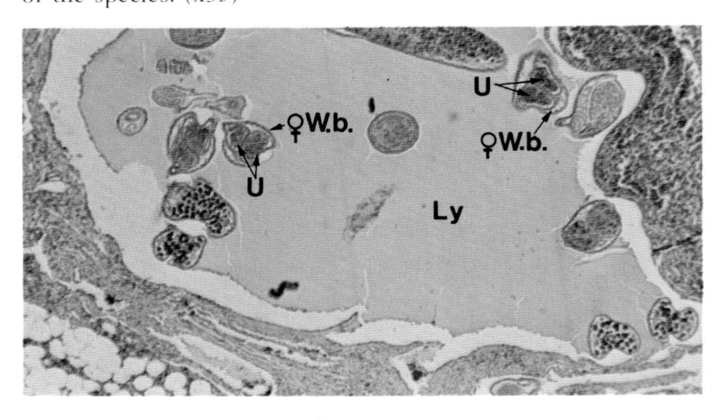

Fig. 107. Wuchereria bancrofti in lymphatic vessel.
This is similar to Figure 106 except no lymphatic fluid is visible within the vessel invaded by *W. bancrofti* (W.b.). However, the wall of the lymphatic vessel still preserves its endothelial lining (End). The parasites in cross-section reveal their characteristic morphology. (U) bilateral uteri. (x35)

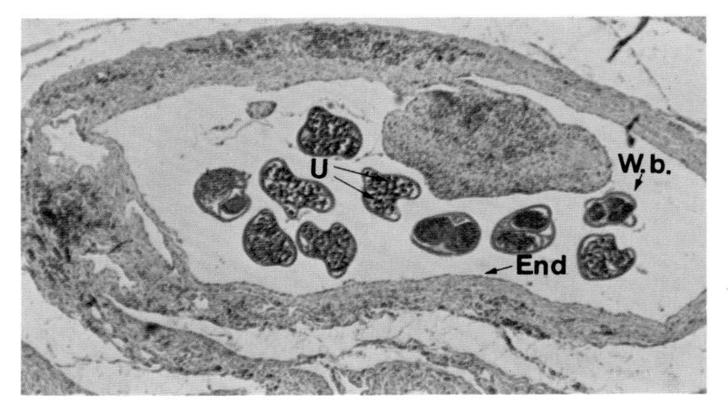

Fig. 108. Wuchereria bancrofti in lymph node.
This is a very old infection with *W. bancrofti* (W.b.). The parasite is calcified and surrounded by collagen tissue (CT) which has replaced the lymphatic vessel. The characteristic paired uteri (U) within the calcified female and its location within the lymphatic system are sufficient for positive diagnosis. (x100)

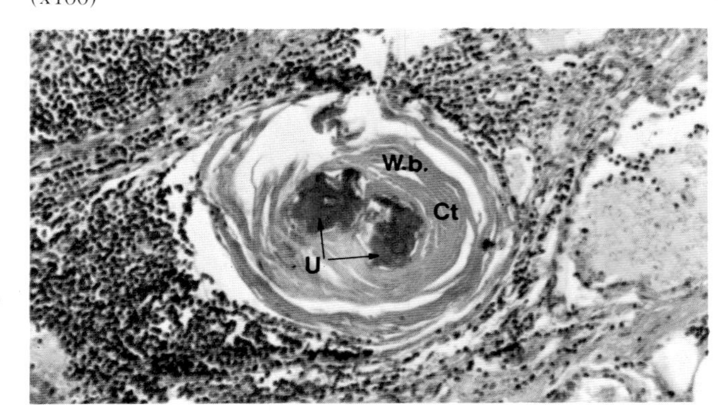

Testes

While the testicle appears to be one of the predilection sites of some infections, e.g., the filtrable virus of mumps, this organ is seldom invaded by parasites.

Except for *W. bancrofti* and aberrant eggs of schistosomes, no parasites are usually found in the testes. In bancroftian filariasis the presence of adult worms is due to the rich lymphatic circulation in this area. The presence of the eggs of blood flukes is purely accidental.

Although the filarial worms of *W. bancrofti* in Africa and South America are morphologically identical, the scrotal elephantiasis is predominantly found in the former location, while elephantiasis of the legs is more frequently observed in the latter endemic area.

Fig. 109. Wuchereria bancrofti in the testis.

An old infection with *W. bancrofti* (W.b.) reveals a few calcified worms within a lymphatic vessel of the testis which has been replaced by collagen tissue. There are two other better preserved worms within the lymphatic plexus. (x40)

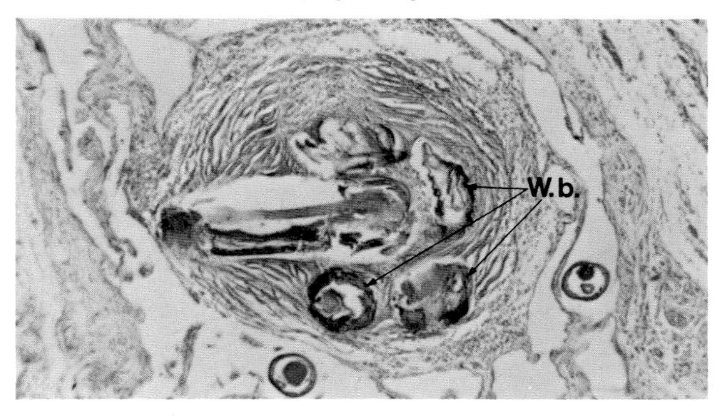

Fig. 110. Schistosoma mansoni ova in the testis.

Cross-section of aberrant eggs (E) of *S. mansoni* in a fibrotic testis (FT). The eggs are diagnostic of the species as two of them reveal long, pointed lateral spines (S). The well rounded outline of these eggs excludes the possibility that these spines are artifacts resulting from cracked, deformed eggshells. (x100)

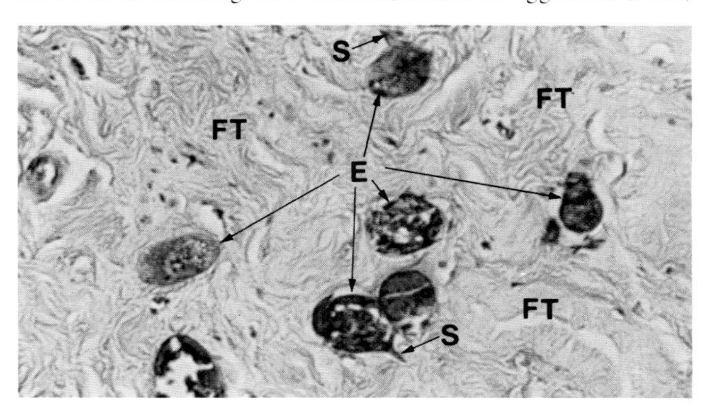

Nervous System

Some parasites show a definite predilection for the nervous system such as the soil-water amebae producing the meningoencephalitis in man. Others affect the brain only in the last stages of the disease, e.g., the trypanosomes of the African sleeping sickness. The nervous system like any other organ may be invaded by aberrant parasites such as the ova of schistosomes, by the larval stages accidentally developing in man, such as *Cysticercus*, or *Echinococcus* cysts. Among the latter group, one accidental parasite of man has a special predilection for the

Fig. 111. Angiostrongylus cantonensis in the brain.
A cross-section of *A. cantonensis* (A.c.) within the meninges, is near a large, congested vessel (CV). Note the holomyerial type of flat, evenly high muscle fibers (MF) under the cuticle (C), and two prominent cords (Cor.). The meninges are infiltrated with eosinophiles and mononuclear cells. (x40)

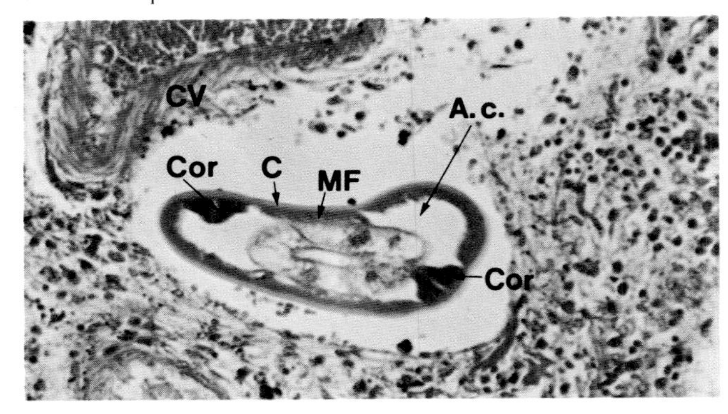

Fig. 112. Trypanosoma rhodesiense.
One identifiable trypanosome (Try), center, in a brain section from a patient with an overwhelming infection due to *T. rhodesiense.* The undulating membrane is not visible but the kinetoplast (K) can be seen to the left of the fusiform protozoon. The absence of reactive changes around the parasite is characteristic of this type of infection. (x1,000)

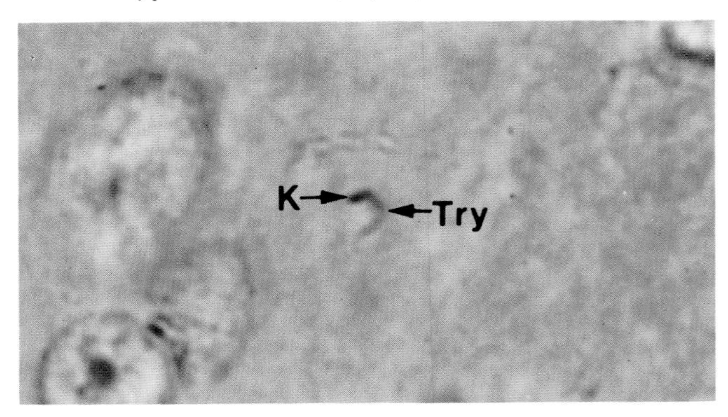

brain during its larval stage. This is *Angiostrongylus cantonensis*, a nematode producing eosinophilic meningoencephalitis.

Angiostrongylus cantonensis

The lung worm of the rat has been found in vast areas of the Far East, including the Pacific islands. The adult parasite measures 7.7-12.8mm., the female being the larger. The intermediate hosts of this parasite are snails, slugs and fresh water shrimps. When a rat gets infected by consuming an intermediate host, the parasitic larvae migrate first to the brain of the rat, where they remain for a short time, and finally move to their usual location in the pulmonary arterioles. In an accidentally infected man, the larvae which migrated to the brain remain there. The damage they cause to the brain is related to their location and their development. Although some infections by *A. cantonensis* in man appear to be self-limited, cases of severe disability and death have been reported. The clinical syndrome produced by this parasite in man is eosinophilic meningoencephalitis.

Trypanosomiasis

The two species of trypanosomes responsible for African sleeping sickness in man are *T. gambiense* and *T. rhodesiense.* Morphologically, the slender, fusiform protozoa, measuring 14-33/1.5-3.5 microns are practically identical. Trypanosomes have an undulating membrane, a nucleus and a terminal kinetoplast. Their intermediate hosts are various species of tsetse flies. *T. gambiense* is limited to tropical West and Central Africa, and *T. rhodesiense* is endemic in East Africa. Clinically, *T. gambiense* is a milder form of trypanosomiasis and may be a self-limited infection. However, the initial vascular and lymphatic stage may progress to the more severe form similar to that observed with *T. rhodesiense.* In the latter, the febrile paroxysms of the early stage, due to multiplication of the trypanosomes, are more severe and more frequent. The final stage of the invasion of the central nervous system comes more regularly and earlier, and frequently assumes a fulminating form. The severity of the neurological disorders depends upon the location of the cerebral lesions. The trypanosomes, which can be observed early in the disease in peripheral blood and lymph nodes, may be found later in various viscera and during the final, cerebral stage in brain sections.

Soil-water amebae

Species of soil-water amebae of the genera *Naegleria* and *Acanthamoeba (Hartmannella)* which for decades were considered nonpathogenic, have been isolated

Fig. 113. Acanthamoeba in the brain.

Two *Acanthamoeba* (A) near the meninges in a case of fatal brain hemorrhage. Both amebae demonstrate typical mottled cytoplasm. The ameba near the eosinophil shows its nucleus (N) with a large dark central karyosome (Kar), but no peripheral chromatin. (x400)

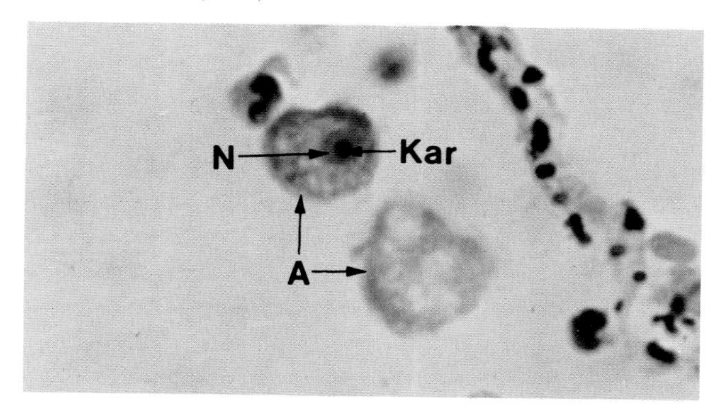

Fig. 114. Acanthamoeba in the brain.

An *Acanthamoeba* (A) surrounded by pus cells (P). The section passes through the nucleus (N) of the ameba demonstrating its typical morphology with a large, central karyosome (Kar) stained dark red and no peripheral chromatin. The cytoplasm is vacuolated. Trichrome (Masson). (x1,000)

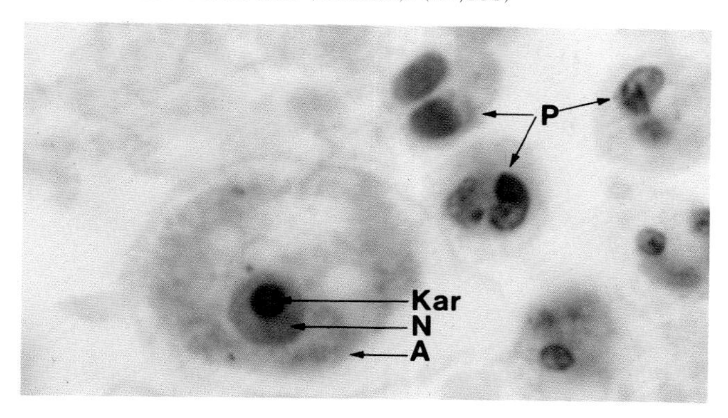

Fig. 115. Cysticercosis. *Cysticercus cellulosae.*

Two larval forms of *T. solium* in brain tissue. One, left, shows the characteristic maze-like folding of *Cysticercus cellulosae* (C.c.). The other, right, shows its empty bladder (B). There is a strong cellular reaction around the cysts. The blood vessel (BV) in the left upper corner is congested. (x25)

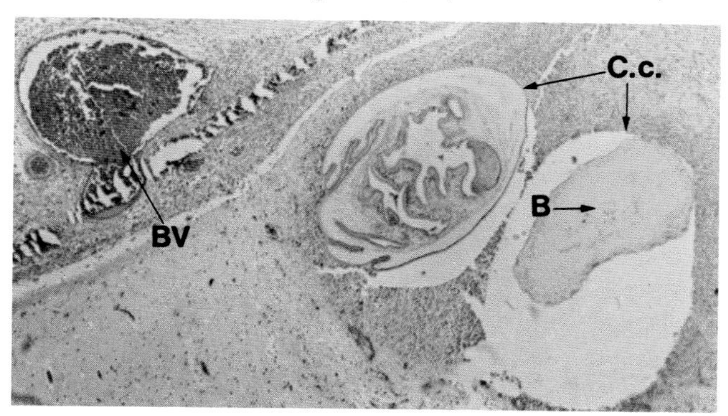

from man in a number of cases, both in Europe and the Americas. These amebae have been found in asymptomatic carriers harboring them in the nasal mucosa but have also been observed in the brains of patients with fulminating meningoencephalitis. Recent observations suggest that the amebae may produce intermediate forms between a carrier stage and a fatal disease and can be harbored in other organs as well. Morphologically, the species of soil-water amebae is difficult to differentiate in tissue sections but this can be done by immunological and cultural methods. Unlike *E. histolytica*, these amebae have a nucleus with a large central karyosome, no peripheral chromatin and the cytoplasm is usually vacuolated. The brain lesions demonstrate congestion or hemorrhages, marked cellular infiltration with both mononuclear and polymorphonuclear cells and also abscess formation.

Fig. 116. Toxoplasmosis. *Toxoplasma gondii* in the brain.

A small group of *T. gondii* (T.g.), center, in a case of congenital toxoplasmosis. The *Toxoplasma* are sectioned at various angles and present a darkly stained nucleus (N) and the absence of a kinetoplast. The parasites sectioned longitudinally show their characteristic crescentic form. There is no cyst formation in this early, acute infection. Giemsa. (x1,000)

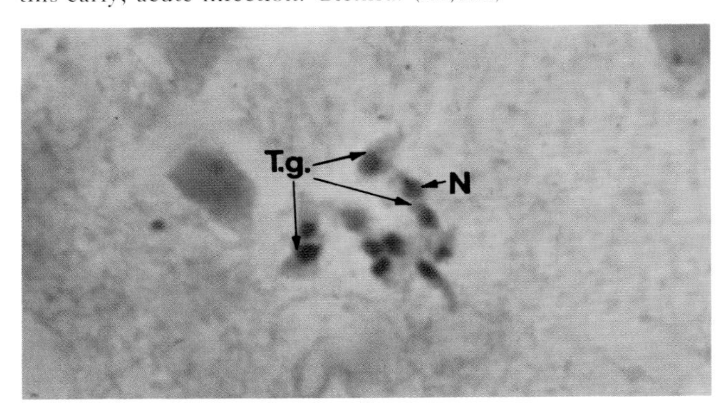

Fig. 117. Malaria. *Plasmodium falciparum* in the brain.

This section of the brain in a case of cerebral malaria demonstrates the typical picture of congested blood vessels. The capillaries contain malarial pigment (P). No parasites of *P. falciparum* can be detected at this magnification. (x100)

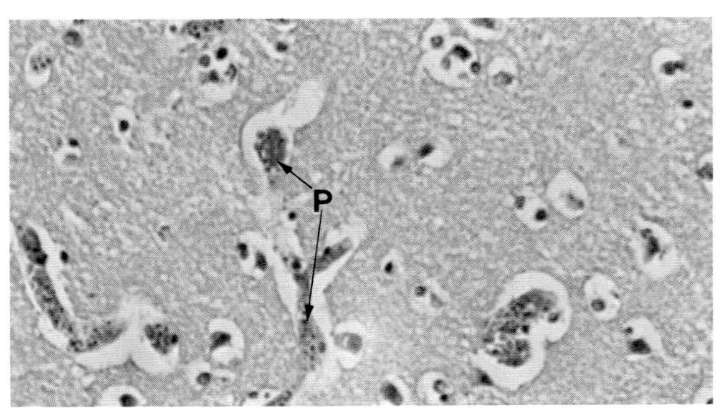

Fig. 118. Schistosomiasis. Ovum of *Schistosoma mansoni* in the spinal cord.

An egg (E) of *S. mansoni*, sectioned lengthwise demonstrating its typical long, lateral spine (S) with a strong tissue reaction around the egg. (x100)

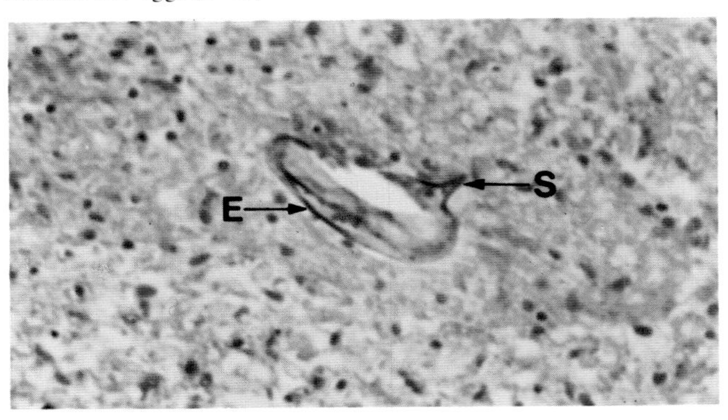

Fig. 119. Visceral larva migrans in the retina.

Part of a visceral larva migrans (VLM) in a longitudinal section, is in a small granuloma (G), within preretinal inflammatory membrane (PIM). (x40)

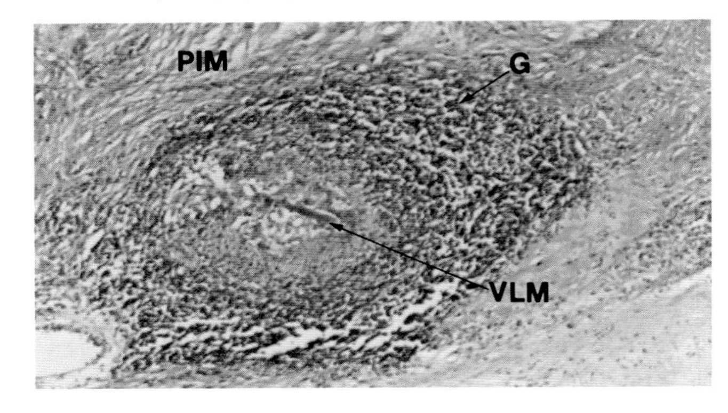

Fig. 120. Visceral larva migrans in the retina.

A visceral larva migrans (VLM), sectioned lengthwise, is in a necrotic area (NA) contained within a preretinal inflammatory membrane (PIM). (x100)

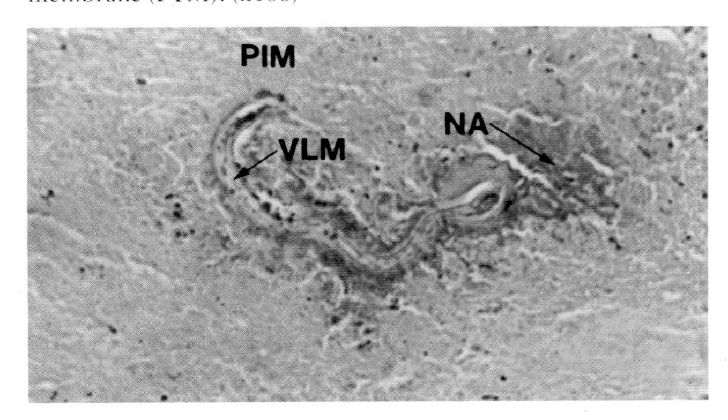